Strong
As a
Mother

Strong
As a
Mother

How to Stay Healthy, Happy, and
(Most Importantly) Sane from
Pregnancy to Parenthood

THE ONLY GUIDE TO TAKING CARE OF *YOU*!

Kate Rope

St. Martin's Griffin
New York

www.stmartins.com

The Library of Congress Cataloging-in-Publication Data
is available upon request.

ISBN 978-1-250-10558-5 (trade paperback)
ISBN 978-1-250-10559-2 (ebook)

Our books may be purchased in bulk for promotional, educational, or business use.
Please contact your local bookseller or the Macmillan Corporate and Premium
Sales Department at 1-800-221-7945, extension 5442, or by email at
MacmillanSpecialMarkets@macmillan.com.

First Edition: May 2018

10 9 8 7 6

This book is dedicated to the WOMEN of the world,
whose mental health should be our top priority.

And to the two STRONG little women who
gave me the opportunity to learn how to
take care of myself as a mom.

And to my HUSBAND, who gave me
the space and time to do it.

And to ME, for doing it.

Contents

Part III: Staying Strong: The Big Picture of Motherhood

Author's Note

I am so glad that you have picked up this book and that you are making your well-being a priority as you begin the adventure of motherhood. It is not an understatement to say that putting your well-being first will make your transition to motherhood so much easier and will be the foundation for a strong, happier family and life as a mom.

I see the transition to motherhood as existing on a spectrum. Everyone struggles in some way, and there are solutions to all those struggles. What kind of support or intervention you need depends on where you fall on the spectrum. For some women, learning how to get good sleep, moving their bodies regularly, and finding good support may be all they need to find their footing and feel strong.

For others who experience perinatal mood or anxiety disorders, such as postpartum depression or anxiety, finding well-trained mental health support can make the difference between struggling every day and beginning to enjoy motherhood. In rare instances, it can be the difference between life and death. I have made every effort to talk honestly and openly about the mental health challenges women are susceptible to at this time of their lives and to include a wide range of expert resources where they can find help.

But I am not a mental health professional, and this book is not a substitute for current medical advice from a health-care provider who can evaluate your particular situation. Any time you are not feeling like yourself or you are suffering, it is vital for your health and your family's health that you reach out for professional support, and if someone you love is not acting like herself or struggling, it is critical that you help get her to medical care.

Just like gestational diabetes, perinatal mood and anxiety disorders are a medical complication of pregnancy for which there is effective, evidenced-based treatment, and the sooner women access it, the sooner they will recover and be ready to take part in this wild, wonderful journey of motherhood. My wish for you is that the compassionate, knowledgeable words of the experts and moms in this book will be the inspiration you need to start feeling better. Because taking care of you is your most important job.

Introduction

Welcome. I am so excited you are here! I can safely say this book is not like any other one you have on your nightstand. It is not a "parenting" book about whether you should let your kid cry it out or have them sleep in the bed next to you. This book is about and for *you*. It is a guide to actually doing what everyone will tell you to do—"take care of yourself"—but no one will show you *how* to do. This book will.

Motherhood is an incredible journey—probably the most life-changing you will ever undertake. It has unimaginable highs and, sometimes, completely unexpected lows. It is the hardest job you will ever love, and it is one where you learn on the job every minute of every day.

New and expecting moms are given buckets of information and advice (some good, some terrible, most unsolicited) about how to give birth to babies and raise children, but few of us receive the focused support and wisdom we need to help *us* adapt to, and thrive in, our new role and new life circumstances. In fact, movies, TV shows, friends, and family often project the image of a seamless transition to motherhood, one in which happiness and confidence come easily.

Yes, there is so much happiness and so many natural moments of wonder ahead, but I don't think there's a mom out there who hasn't struggled through an equal (or greater) number of times when she was unsure of what she was doing, felt overwhelmed by the challenges before her, was too exhausted to think straight, wondered where some part of her had gone to, or just wanted to feel supported, understood, and accepted through all of it.

ALL MOMS ARE WELCOME HERE

Whatever your point of embarkation—pregnancy, adoption, third-party reproduction, or another way—whatever your family looks like—a mom and a dad, two moms, just you, or another configuration—whatever background or community you come from, whatever challenges you face, this book is for you.

We are all human beings, and we will have different and complicated reactions to different phases and experiences of pregnancy and parenthood. That is not only okay, it is beautiful. It would be so boring if we were all the same.

HOW TO USE THIS BOOK

Think of it as a nonjudgmental friend who is willing to listen to everything—the good, the bad, and the ugly—and who is committed to lifting you up when you are down, celebrating with you when you are excited, researching the best ways to get you safely over the bumps on the road, and making sure that you really, truly are taking care of yourself. The book is divided into three parts:

Part I: Expecting Strong: Your Emotional Guide to
  Pregnancy
Part II: Starting Strong: Your Guide to Thriving in the
  First Year
Part III: Staying Strong: The Big Picture of
  Motherhood

CHOOSE YOUR OWN ADVENTURE

Part I: For those opening this book before—or in the early part of—pregnancy, you might want to read straight through.

Part II: If you're picking this book up after pregnancy or you are a non-bio or adoptive mom, this is likely where you'll want to begin. It tackles big topics that apply all the way through motherhood—such as how to get good sleep for your mental health, ways to make exercise and self-care a habit, how to manage conflict with your partner, sex, mental health disorders and how to get help for them, returning to work, and much more.

Part III the final section, covers the philosophical issues of motherhood, including the historical and current expectations placed on mothers and how they shape the way we treat ourselves as mothers and people. But it also has very practical advice for approaching the job as a learning experience, being kind to yourself when things go differently from how you'd wanted, letting go of the urge to compare yourself to others, and why being a "good enough mother" is the best possible thing you can do for your family and yourself.

Within each part are clearly named sections that will tell you exactly the issues they address, such as:

"Why Sleep Matters and How to Get It"
"Preparing to Feed Your Child in a Way That Works
    for You"
"Sex During Pregnancy"
"Bonding with Babies 101"

So, you can also pop in and out of the sections that speak to wherever you are on the journey.

I promise that somewhere in this book you will find a challenge (or twenty-three) you are facing (or have faced) and concrete ways to move through it and arrive at a stronger place.

EXPERT ADVICE

I have woven my personal story into this book, because it is the reason I knew it had to be written, but I spoke with more than one hundred experts who spend all their time researching pregnancy, motherhood, emotional health, and more to offer you scientifically validated solutions and support.

Here's a short list of the kinds of experts I spoke with:

- sleep
- exercise
- genetic testing

- social support
- grief
- sex
- relationships
- parenting
- birth
- infant development
- maternal and reproductive mental health
- feeding (both breast and formula)
- childcare
- career coaching
- self-compassion
- self-care
- motherhood historians and psychologists

READ THE VOICES OF OTHER MOMS IN THE "BEEN THERE, DONE THAT" SECTIONS

All our experiences are unique to us, but I can guarantee that there is another woman out there who has felt or feels very similar to how you are feeling. That's why I surveyed nearly two hundred women from around the country and even a few overseas to include their voices, experiences, and advice in the "Been There, Done That" sections. I am so grateful for the honesty and detail they brought to their answers.

I think of those sections as sitting down with an incredibly diverse and nonjudgmental moms' group where everyone feels free to say just what she is going through. I know they will bring you relief, camaraderie, humor, and some really good advice that can only come from people who have been there and done that.

MY GREAT HOPE

My goal for this book is to give you tools to build for yourself a supportive community and a strong base from which to launch the greatest adventure of your life. It is adaptable and heterogeneous. The only uniform message I have to share is that becoming a parent is likely the most profound experience you will have in your lifetime, and no experience worth its life-changing salt will be easy. There will be struggle. There will be lows. There will be highs. And long stretches in between that feel monotonous when you are in them but may prove beautiful when you look back at them.

And when you struggle, and when it's hard, you should have license to express that, to reach out for help, to try something new, and find a way forward that is easier for you. You should feel supported through all of this. You deserve to have whatever you need to be *strong as a mother*.

You ready?

Expecting Strong

*Your Emotional Guide
to Pregnancy*

You're Pregnant, Now What?

Few things are as profound as looking down at a pregnancy test and seeing that second line slowly appear, and any emotional response you have to big news like this is completely acceptable. You might feel shock, glee, fear, deep satisfaction, relief, panic, incredible joy. You might shriek. You might cry. You might shout a joyful expletive. You might cuss in despair. You might just stare mutely in disbelief.

Maybe you've been trying for a long time and are used to seeing a blank space where that faint marker now appears. Maybe you just started trying and didn't expect to hit the jackpot right away. Or maybe you weren't trying at all and the news is not only unexpected but maybe not even welcomed. You may cycle through ten different emotions as your mind works to wrap itself around the news. Allow yourself to feel whatever comes up for you, and don't judge yourself for it. You're human. This is big news. However you respond is okay.

GIVE YOURSELF TIME TO LET THE NEWS—AND FEELINGS—SINK IN

However you feel as you consider what you have ahead of you, take time for yourself to settle into this new experience. Soon enough you will be swept into planning and decision-making. Take this time to celebrate. If the news arrives to mixed emotions, take some time to see what comes up for you. Maybe write down what you are feeling, or find a friend you can say anything to and tell her everything that comes to mind. Put it all out there. Take a look at what you're feeling and sit with those emotions. If this information represents an abrupt change of plans, give yourself the space to grapple with how you feel and how you want to move forward.

The bottom line is that no matter how you came to those two lines, many different experiences and choices will flow from it. Take as long as you need to sit with the news and see how the news sits with you. Learning to take a pause in the face of what may feel like impending chaos is a skill that will serve you throughout motherhood. Take a moment for you.

When you're ready, read on for guidance on managing the unexpected emotions of pregnancy, weathering the anxieties of the first trimester and beyond, strengthening your relationship with your partner, and learning how you can begin to take care of yourself *now* so you know how to do it well when your world changes.

Been There, Done That: Moms Share the Feelings They Had When They Found Out They Were Pregnant

Panic. Shock. For the first time in my life, I felt like, "I can't control this journey at all. I'm on the roller coaster now, just hold tight."   —RACHEL, LONDON, UK

Absolute joy. It was a difficult journey trying to get pregnant.   —ERICA, STATE COLLEGE, PENNSYLVANIA

I was excited and terrified. Then I realized I'd have to actually give birth and had a panic attack.
    —BECKY, DECATUR, GEORGIA

I was terrified, and I felt guilty for not wanting to be pregnant. So many of my friends were trying for babies, but we, who had never wanted children of our own, had accidentally gotten pregnant.   —EMILY T.

Terrified, elated, and everything in between.
    —ALEXIS, SAINT PAUL, MINNESOTA

I was happy, but also pretty confused by it. I felt pretty aware I didn't actually know yet what was happening or how my life was going to change.
    —LAUREL, ATLANTA, GEORGIA

It's Natural to Worry: Anxiety in Early Pregnancy

Pregnancy launches you into the responsibility of parenthood—caring for another human life, and that is going to be scary at times (okay, maybe a lot of the time). Worrying will come with the territory, and one of the first places you may feel that concern is over miscarriage.

The reality is that as many as one in four pregnancies end in miscarriage. So it makes sense that women in the early weeks of pregnancy often spend some (or a lot of) time worrying about it. In fact, with technology to detect pregnancies before we even miss a period, we are learning we are pregnant earlier than ever and spending a longer period of time in a kind of early pregnancy limbo.

"We are born with millions and millions of eggs, which means that some won't be able to develop into full pregnancy, and our bodies know what to do with them," says Lauren Abrams, CNM, director of midwifery at Mount Sinai Hospital in Manhattan. "It can be devastating emotionally, but it's not abnormal and, in most cases, does not in any way mean you won't carry a pregnancy to full term." But waiting out those first seven to eight weeks, when the chance of miscarriage is highest, can feel like being on pins and needles.

THE DIMMER SWITCH

My husband was surprised when our first pregnancy didn't feel like an all-or-nothing proposition but rather like a "dimmer switch" that slowly brightened with each passing week and doctor's appointment—until we felt comfortable looking ahead with relative security. The point at which women feel confident in their pregnancies is different for different people.

Some may feel confident and future-focused from the moment they get the news. Others may not count their chicken until twelve weeks. And, for others, it may take longer, especially if they have experienced a pregnancy loss in the past (see "What If I Have Had a Pregnancy Loss Before?" pages 16–17) or are experiencing confusing symptoms. Wherever you fall on that continuum, know that you are not alone.

"It's totally normal, if uncomfortable," says Sarah Best, LCSW, a psychotherapist in New York City who specializes in reproductive mental health. Each visit to the doctor—for your first ultrasound or to hear the baby's heartbeat—can feel like a hurdle to overcome on the road to feeling confident in your pregnancy. A lot of women "feel a little worried and a little hopeful every time they go," says Best.

If your level of concern is not interfering with your life and you are able to enjoy a little bit of fantasizing about what your life will be like with your new baby, Best recommends "riding that wave of worry" and doing what you can to take care of yourself (see page 50) in those early weeks. "Think about if a friend were in a similar situation," advises Best. "How would you offer her support?"

··

Ways to Manage Anxiety During Early Pregnancy

··

Experts will tell you that trying to wish anxious thoughts away will only make them stick around longer, so one approach is to acknowledge the thought you are having, accept that it is okay, and then move forward with some activities that will help you focus on the present moment you are in, rather than the imagined future in your head.

Best recommends taking a break from anxious thoughts by doing activities that involve coordination of your body and mind, such as:

- Crossword puzzles
- Painting
- Adult coloring books
- Sudoku
- Cooking from a recipe
- Yoga
- Walking with a friend
- Gardening
- Meditation
- Mindfulness exercises

"Anything that helps a woman get out of her own head is going to be a good choice," recommends Best.

What If I Have Had a Pregnancy Loss Before?

If you have experienced a pregnancy loss in the past— miscarriage or stillbirth—then the way you feel during this current pregnancy is likely to be very different from someone who is pregnant for the first time. At the Seleni Institute, where I work as editorial director, there is an amazing grief therapist, Christiane Manzella, PhD, who has a compassionate and honest approach to supporting patients through loss.

"I expect to see anxiety," says Manzella, "because their uncertainty is now heightened and uncertainty is one of the most difficult things for people to tolerate in life." And while part of the recovery from your previous loss can be pregnancy and a live birth, Manzella says that "neither is a fix for anguish and anxiety."

What can help is "talking with somebody who is able to listen to you and be present with you while you describe what you are going through. When you are able to talk and be heard, you are moving through your grief, not moving on. You've changed. You've lost some of your innocence, and this pregnancy may not have the warm fuzzies you may have had with your first." You may have lost the ability to see the birth of a baby as an inevitable end to your pregnancy journey, and that is expected, says Manzella.

Find someone with whom you feel comfortable and talk about what you are feeling and what has helped you in moments of anxiety in the past. Do you want people to just listen to what you are feeling? Do you want suggestions of what could help? If your current pregnancy allows, can you do some consistent mild exercise? Does listening to music help you? Would having a regular lunch with your supportive friend give you something to look forward to and a space where you know all your thoughts and feelings can be safely shared?

The professional support of a therapist, like Manzella, who is trained in grief and perinatal loss or reproductive mental health can be a tremendous support, especially if you find that your distress is intense. See page 368 for places to find one. "Reach out," says Manzella. "There is no reason for you to suffer alone." And you are not alone. Many women have been—and are—where you sit now. See "Been There, Done That."

BEWARE THE GOOGLE TRAP

"You are never going to get straight answers from Google. There is going to be conflicting information even from reliable sources," warns Best. "A lot of the moms I work with will be experiencing some symptom—cramping, spotting, something—and they end up on a five-year-old message board with very extreme personal accounts that don't have happy endings. They might find a lot of stories with happy endings too, but the thing about humans is that we tend to dismiss the positives and assume that the one negative thing we read is the more likely outcome."

In general, information seeking, like repeatedly typing your symptoms into Google, usually heightens anxiety rather than alleviating it. "It's like scratching a mosquito bite," explains Best. "When the results come up, at first you feel some relief, but it's short-lived, and then the stress is there again.

There is always the thought, 'If I just get some piece of information, this worry will go away,' but the reality is the information rarely makes it go away; it just reinforces the idea that you should keep looking for information."

DR. GOOGLE IS NOT A MEDICAL PROFESSIONAL— YOUR PROVIDER IS

"The best thing a woman can do in that early period is to develop a relationship with her care provider," says Best. "If you don't feel comfortable talking about these concerns with your OB or midwife, the first trimester is an excellent time to transfer to a provider with whom you are more comfortable." Once you feel comfortable with your health-care provider, rely on him or her in times of concern. Only he or she knows your specific situation and can speak to it with authority. "True information from a care provider familiar with your case can be an excellent balm," advises Best.

What If I Lose My Pregnancy While I Am Reading This Book?

If you have a pregnancy loss, first know that I am so, so sorry and wish I could be there to listen to everything you are feeling right now, and I hope you have a good friend or family member who can do that for you.

It's probably time for you to put this book back up on your shelf until it makes sense for you to take it down again, but before you do, let me offer some advice from grief specialist Christiane Manzella, PhD.

"Grief is a process that people move through," says Manzella. "During it, you will feel many feelings and thoughts—unexpected and expected—and sometimes you will have thoughts that seem crazy to you, and you may feel many different things at once. You may also experience physical sensations (and your body might be lactating or bleeding)." Manzella recommends first and foremost "making sure you eat, sleep, and get good support from your friends and loved ones."

It's also important to understand that if you are experiencing grief, it is real. Perinatal loss often goes unrecognized and unsupported. There are no mourning rituals for pregnancy loss—especially miscarriage. There are no culturally developed scripts to help people know what to say or do.

Which means that often even the people in your immediate family won't understand how you are feeling. They may think or say things like "What's wrong with her?" "When will she get over it?" or "You're young; you can have another." But if you are grieving, there is no "getting over" it; there is only moving through it. When you can give voice to what you are experiencing and feeling, says Manzella, "that is how you move through it."

Consider reaching out to a professional who specializes in perinatal loss. "Do it earlier than later," says Manzella, "just to have someone who understands the process of perinatal loss listen to you and help you move through grief in a way that is more adaptive and will help you to keep from getting stuck. Women do move through this."

There are more resources for getting the support you need on page 373. I recommend making use of them, as well as your most understanding friends and family, until you are ready to pick this book up again. It will be here if—or when—you are.

HOW DO I KNOW IF I NEED HELP
WITH MY ANXIETY?

If your worry starts to affect your day-to-day life—keeping you from sleeping or eating, functioning as you normally would, or enjoying your life—or if you find it hard to balance your concerns with a little optimism and constantly assume the worst is going to happen, Best recommends checking in with your obstetrician or a mental health professional who specializes in reproductive health (see page 38 for more about anxiety in pregnancy). He or she can help assess whether you are experiencing anxiety that could benefit from treatment (which can be psychotherapy or medication or a combination of the two).

The first nine weeks of my second pregnancy were an anxiety-filled ride. I went to weekly therapy sessions and talked extensively with my obstetrician about the possibility that I might need to return to the antidepressant I had used for postpartum anxiety after my first daughter was born. But at nine weeks, the anxiety dissipated, and I entered a more hopeful, forward-facing stage of pregnancy.

The most important thing is getting the support you need until that happens for you.

Managing Anxiety Around Genetic Testing

One of the amazing parts of modern pregnancy is what we are able to learn about our developing babies. It can be incredibly helpful and comforting. But the amount of information can also be overwhelming and cause unnecessary anxiety. Psychologists will tell you that making decisions is one of the greatest sources of stress we face in life, and you are about to make a lot of them.

Find Out Your Choices

Ask your doctor or midwife what tests are routinely offered by their practice. Broadly speaking, there are two kinds of tests—screening tests and diagnostic tests. Screening tests cannot tell you whether your baby does—or does not—have a particular condition. These tests can only determine whether you have an *increased risk* of having a baby with a particular condition. Diagnostic tests, which are invasive—meaning that a needle is inserted into your womb to gather genetic information—can confirm whether your baby has a medical condition. Because they are invasive, they carry a small risk of miscarriage.

Ask What Information the Tests Can Provide

Before you say yes to a particular test, it's important to know what you will learn from the test and what you think you will do with the information. One of the reasons this is important is that, especially with screening tests, the results can sound scary even when they are not.

"There is not a 'yes' or 'no' answer in a screening test," explains Katie Stoll, MS, LGC, director of clinical services at the Genetic Support Foundation in Olympia, Washington, "just a higher or lower chance that your baby has a particular condition." And even an increased chance can still be a very remote one. It's also very important to find out how often the screening test can produce a false positive, meaning the test indicates you have a higher risk of having a child with a particular condition when she does not. Most practices have a genetic counselor you can consult if you have an abnormal result or are considering an invasive test.

Find Out Your Baseline Risk

The counselor or your doctor can tell you your risk of having a baby with a condition such as Down syndrome based on the age you will be when your baby is due. "Many women are low risk and will find reassurance by just learning what the probability is to begin with," says Stoll. If your baseline risk feels comfortable to you, you may decide not to screen for the condition.

Ask Yourself (and Your Partner): Why Do I/We Want to Know?

Most of the time when we take these tests, we are just hoping to hear that everything is going to be okay. But the problem is that these tests can have false positives and abnormal results, so it's a really good idea to think about how you might feel and the steps you would take if you get worrisome or inconclusive information.

Put Things in Perspective

If you learn that you have a 1 percent chance that your child will be born with Down syndrome, that means that "the chance your baby does not have Down syndrome is 99 percent," explains Jill Fonda, a prenatal genetic counselor with Maternal Fetal Medicine and Genetics of the Medical Faculty Associates (MFA) at George Washington University in Washington, DC. "So write 99 percent down and hang it on your refrigerator."

Realize There Is No Perfect Decision

When Fonda talks to couples about making these choices, she tries to help them understand that "there may not be a perfect decision about testing. They have to make the best choice for them." And that advice applies to so much in this book!

Been There, Done That: Moms Share Their Fears in Early Pregnancy and How They Managed Them

---

I worried about how my future child would turn out. Keeping a pregnancy journal helped improve my mood by allowing me to sort out the "stories" from fact.

—SARA, ATLANTA, GEORGIA

I was always worried there was something wrong. I am an older mother, and my second was conceived by IVF. It helped to go to my doctor appointments, and yoga helped a lot. I told myself when the thoughts crept in that the majority of pregnancies result in a healthy baby.

—MOM TO TWO IN DECATUR, GEORGIA

With both my children, my primary feeling was anxiety at the beginning, because I had miscarried prior pregnancies. Relaxation exercises and tapes and psychotherapy helped me cope. I talked to friends who had miscarried and understood my fears. I knew I couldn't remove the fear and just had to live through it. I also prayed and went to church.

—COLLEEN, BROOKLYN, NEW YORK

I worried about my ability to be a mum. How the baby would impact my relationship with my husband. Whether we would have much sex again and how we would cope with the changes. Therapy helped.

—RACHEL, LONDON, UK

When Should I Spill the Beans?

A common threshold for sharing the news is twelve weeks, once the risk of miscarriage has significantly decreased and when you may begin to show. But there's no rule about when to spill the beans. Reflect on how you have coped with emotionally significant moments in the past (and whether it worked for you) to think through how you want to approach sharing your news now.

Would you like to talk about what you are going through and get support from other people? Or do you prefer to keep things to yourself and talk about them once you have sorted through your own feelings on the topic? When something difficult or exciting happens, do you want to hop on the phone to your best friend? Or do you want to retreat to your couch for a while to let things soak in privately?

It's also useful to think about whether you will want support when you get ultrasound results, if something concerning happens with the pregnancy, or if you experience significant nausea and/or vomiting. If your mom will be a good support through times like that, then you will want her to know earlier.

On the other hand, if your sister likes to hash out worst-case scenarios more likely to cause you anxiety, it's fine for her to wait to get the news. What will make you (and your partner) most comfortable?

Some Reasons to Share
- You rely heavily on emotional support from friends and family
- You are having significant nausea and/or vomiting and need practical and emotional support
- Sharing the news with others will help you feel engaged and optimistic about the pregnancy
- If something unexpected happens, you would want people there to support you through it

Some Reasons to Wait
- You value privacy when it comes to life changes
- You want to receive genetic resting results and make choices based on that information in private
- If something unexpected happens, you would rather work through it on your own or with your partner

"You aren't obligated to tell your mom, let alone your mother-in-law, about your pregnancy status," says Paula Spencer Scott, a pregnancy etiquette expert and author of *Momfidence!: An Oreo Never Killed Anybody and Other Secrets to Happier Parenting*. "Don't get goaded into it before you're ready." If someone puts you in a tight spot (like asking whether you turned down that glass of wine for "a reason"), you will be forgiven a little white lie, such as "I'm just not feeling well" or "I'm on antibiotics." Or you can be more direct and let the person know that you appreciate their interest and assure them that when you have news to share, they will be among the first to know.

There is no right or wrong way or time to share your news. What matters is that you feel comfortable doing so. Talk through the options with your partner. If, later, someone expresses hurt that you did not tell them "soon enough," you will be able to explain simply why it mattered to you to wait, and most people will understand. If they don't, well, then it's likely there's no way you could have done it "right" to satisfy them, and this moment is about you and the family you are building.

Been There, Done That: Moms' Tales of Sharing Their News

I never subscribed to the notion of not telling people. If they were in my life, then they knew there was something seriously wrong with me, because I had hyperemesis gravidarum (severe nausea and vomiting during pregnancy), and if/when I had an issue with the pregnancies, I needed the whole village to rally.

—ERICA, PITTSBURGH, PENNSYLVANIA

I remember being a little worried, and a friend asked me if I was filled with joy. I told her I was. She said, "Then why not share that as long as you have it? You shouldn't have to suppress the joy now for the fear of the unknown." I took that to heart.

—AMANDA, PORTLAND, OREGON

My husband and I agreed to wait twelve weeks before telling anyone, out of an abundance of caution and just to avoid the potentially uncomfortable conversation of explaining a miscarriage. This worked well for us and allowed us time to enjoy a little "secret" together.   —Rebecca

I told people right away. I'm not one to hold back, and if I were to lose the pregnancy, the people in my life are my greatest support.   —Nicole, Brooklyn, New York

What Was That?! The Unexpected Emotions of Pregnancy

We are human beings. We have complicated emotions. That's normal, and pregnancy is no different. You may feel elated, scared, overwhelmed, disbelieving, regretful, resentful, euphoric, jealous. There are a million ways to respond to this radical change in your life, and that's expected. But you may not *feel* like it's okay to feel anything but unremitting joy when everyone is congratulating you and focusing on how thrilled you must be. I'm here to tell you that all your feelings are valid (and mental health experts back me up on this), and if some of them feel a little off the popular pregnancy script, you are in great company (see "Been There, Done That," page 32).

"Human beings have an amazing capacity to hold multiple emotions at the same time," says New York City therapist Sarah Best, LCSW. "We are masters of ambivalence." The important thing to remember as you move through your pregnancy (and through parenthood, for that matter) is that "when it comes to mental health, there's no such thing as a good or bad emotion," says Best. "Feelings are just information that tells us what's happening for us and gives us clues about how we need to care for ourselves."

If you are experiencing emotions you didn't expect to have during pregnancy, the first step is to acknowledge them. If you can do that without judging yourself, you will give yourself the emotional space to address them and figure out what you need. If, on the other hand, you try to suppress or ignore the emotions you are feeling, because you don't think you "should" feel the way you do, you will likely find them growing stronger or expressing themselves in unpleasant ways.

. . . .

Ways to Manage Difficult Emotions in Pregnancy

. . . .

- Be kind to yourself (see page 335 for self-compassion exercises).
- Spend time with friends.
- Share your feelings with someone you trust.
- Know that things will change and you will not feel this way forever.
- Think about how you would support a friend who was feeling the way you are. What would you tell her? Tell that to yourself. Write it down if it helps you believe it or so you can refer back to it.
- If you feel really stuck in a particular feeling, such as anger or anxiety, consider reaching out to a mental health professional to get some support working through your emotions. (See page 38 for information on mood and anxiety disorders during pregnancy.)

Having complicated emotional responses to being pregnant does not mean that you won't be a good mom or that you don't love your baby or that you are not grateful to be pregnant. It just means you're a human expecting a big life change (all while hormones rise and fall in your body in large amounts) and you are going to have a lot of feelings about it. End of story. Okay, really beginning of story. Read on.

What If I Don't Feel Bonded to My Developing Baby?

Some women immediately feel a connection to the life developing inside them. For others, the idea of a living being growing inside of them can feel downright "creepy," says Sarah Best, LCSW. "And that's totally fine. It *is* kind of a creepy thing. You have sex with someone, and then something starts growing in your body and then you push it out of your vagina. That's crazy!"

"I talk to so many moms who feel like, 'I have an alien growing inside me,'" says Margaret Howard, PhD, professor of psychiatry and human behavior and medicine at the Alpert Medical School of Brown University in Providence, Rhode Island. "But they are taking good care of the baby, and that's totally within the spectrum of normal."

"We are wired to bond with our babies, without doing it in an intentional way," says Best. "Attachment happens. I'm more concerned about somebody being critical of themselves when they don't feel blissed out."

There could be times when the intensity of your feelings indicates that you might be experiencing a mood disorder—such as depression or anxiety (see pages 38–47)—and will feel better with professional support. If you are feeling unremitting anger or hate toward your baby or you are consumed with worry about the feelings you are having about your baby, Best says it is important to talk with a mental health professional who can help you sort through your feelings and come to a better place. (See page 367 to help you find one.)

Been There, Done That: Moms Share Unexpected Feelings During Pregnancy

---

I didn't enjoy being pregnant, and that was a surprise to me. Not everyone feels energized and glowing from the experience. It is what it is—different for everyone—and it has no bearing on what kind of mother you'll be.

—Nicole, Brooklyn, New York

I anticipated liking being pregnant, but I didn't anticipate loving every minute—good, bad, and ugly—as much as I did. —Betsy, Atlanta, Georgia

In the beginning, I didn't feel a connection and was sad about that. Once I felt the kicks, it all changed for me. —Kym

I felt bonded, but in an abstract way, nothing like after she was born. It was weird that I had something growing inside me but not as weird as it was cool.

—Stephanie, Illinois

For some women, pregnancy feels like the ultimate test of emotional/psychological endurance and strength and not

*like butterflies and warm breezes and constant reassuring
kicks from the baby. There's often a mix and plenty of ups
and downs and ambivalence. It's okay to not feel joyous or
especially strong all the time. That was my "normal" experience of pregnancy, and I'm increasingly aware that I was
not alone.*   —DIANA, MONTCLAIR, NEW JERSEY

*I was taken aback with my second by how disappointed I
was at twenty weeks to learn I was having a second boy. It
took me months to recover.*   —ANONYMOUS

*I found it difficult for the first half of pregnancy to meet
people's excitement. "Are you* so *excited?" was a tough question for me to answer. Having a child has been framed as
the very best, most wonderful thing, yet we know that it's
infinitely more complex than that.*

—EMILY, ATLANTA, GEORGIA

Am I a Terrible Mother If I Have a Cup of Coffee?

As soon as you find out you are pregnant, you are made keenly aware of a list of rules you are expected to follow. Alcohol is out. So are cigarettes. So is unpasteurized cheese and deli meat. Sushi's off the table, and you have to start checking the linings on those cans of fiber-filled beans you're supposed to eat to make sure you steer clear of BPA. Then there are the things you should be doing: taking prenatal vitamins, eating fish (but the *right* kind of fish) for healthy brain development, exercising (but doing the *right* kind of exercise, with permission from your doctor), and so on.

It can seem exciting to know that you are doing something so important that there are rules you are expected to follow. But there's also a downside: it can make you feel that every choice you make has the potential to either boost your child's chance of getting into college or threaten his very existence. And—with few exceptions—neither is true.

GETTING PERSPECTIVE

When Emily Oster, Ph.D., professor of economics at Brown University in Providence, Rhode Island, was pregnant with her first child, she felt frustrated by the lack of research-based information about all the rules she faced, so she decided to evaluate the data herself. She read thousands of medical papers, looking for the best information about what she should really be worried about.

And this is what she learned: some of the rules (no excessive drinking, taking folic acid, avoiding contact sports and skiing) are absolutely backed up by good data. Others, like the prohibition against deli meat and caffeine, not as much. So she wrote a book, *Expecting Better: Why the Conventional Medical Wisdom Is Wrong—and What You Really Need to Know*, that would help women make choices in pregnancy based on good science.

The trouble with "these rules," according to Oster, "is that they have gotten turned into a commentary on how much you value your baby. You think, *If I am able to deny myself this thing that I like, then it shows how good a mom I will be.*"

"All of the emphasis on the things you can do or not do during pregnancy for your child's well-being leads to a culture of success or failure around your fetus," says Mara Acel-Green, MSW, a psychotherapist who specializes in maternal mental health and is the owner of Strong Roots Counseling in Boston, Massachusetts. "What you eat, how you behave, it's all on you."

HOW TO FEEL GOOD ABOUT THE CHOICES YOU MAKE IN PREGNANCY

One way to tackle the rules, says Acel-Green, is to think about what you *can* eat and what you *can* do instead of what you can't. Make a list of your favorite foods and indulgences that you are encouraged to enjoy during pregnancy. Then shop for those things and have them on hand so you can feel like you are enjoying yourself at the same time as you are making choices you feel good about for your baby.

Evaluating your choices is also an opportunity to let go of a little control (a skill parenthood forces you to practice time and again). The reality is that we do not—nor will we ever— have complete power over how our children develop or who they become (and accepting that fact is both scary and liberating). Yes, we can do things in pregnancy that are proven to be good for our children's health—like taking folic acid and avoiding cigarettes and excessive alcohol. But these are changes that benefit us as well, and they give us an opportunity to frame pregnancy as a moment to take care of ourselves.

Been There, Done That: Moms Share How They Felt About the Rules of Pregnancy

---

I waited for my husband to come home and smoked my last-ever cigarette while telling him. That was probably the greatest part in the beginning—knowing I could finally let go of that addiction, that my body had a greater purpose. I still remember July 25, 2009, as the day I quit smoking instead of the day I found out I was pregnant with my first child. —AMANDA, PORTLAND, OREGON

Following the rules felt like something I could do to give me a tiny measure of control in the situation. Giving up drinking for nine months seemed a small price to pay.

—COLLEEN, BROOKLYN, NEW YORK

Not drinking was the hardest. I didn't realize how much I relied on that glass of wine or beer after work to relax.

—MOM TO A TODDLER IN NORTH CAROLINA

I thought a lot of it was moralizing, so I sought out science-backed websites that actually investigated the restrictions. I followed the ones that had evidence to back them up and ignored the others. —STEPHANIE, ILLINOIS

If you listen to everything that you are and are not supposed to eat while pregnant, you'd starve! Just eat. Be healthy. Enjoy it! —DOMINGA, SAINT PAUL, MINNESOTA

What If This Doesn't Feel Like "The Happiest Time of My Life"?

We've already covered a lot of the very understandable and common emotions you can experience during pregnancy. If you find that reading this book, talking things through with good friends, and/or employing some techniques for self-care help you manage difficult feelings, great. If you don't, if your concerns are growing or you find it difficult to function relatively comfortably most days, then you may be experiencing what the experts call a perinatal mood or anxiety disorder (PMAD).

What used to be called *postpartum depression* is now understood to be a spectrum of conditions that can develop during pregnancy and in the first year of motherhood. These conditions are common and treatable and nothing to be ashamed of. In fact, PMADs are among the *most common* complications of pregnancy.

"About 15 percent of women will have depression during pregnancy," says Ruta Nonacs, MD, staff psychiatrist at the Center for Women's Mental Health at Massachusetts General Hospital in Boston and editor of Womensmentalhealth .org. That's almost twice the percentage of women who will develop gestational diabetes, and yet, unlike diabetes, women are not routinely screened for mood disorders in pregnancy.

"Depression has been under-recognized in pregnant women," says Margaret Howard, PhD. "And a lot of that is because so many women chalk up their symptoms of depression to being pregnant." And women may even be less aware when they are experiencing anxiety, which some research suggests is more common in pregnancy.

"Anxiety symptoms often co-occur with mood symptoms in the perinatal period," says Samantha Meltzer-Brody, MD, director of the perinatal psychiatry program at the UNC Center for Women's Mood Disorders in Chapel Hill, North Carolina. "For some women, normal worries about the pregnancy start to become persistent and can feel overwhelming. This often also corresponds with lower mood or feeling less enjoyment in usual activities."

Whether you entered pregnancy with a mental health diagnosis or start to feel badly during pregnancy, you have nothing to be ashamed of. The way you feel is no indication of how much you love your baby, what kind of mom you will be, or the kind of person you are. PMADs are just something that can happen when you mix a major life transition with tectonic shifts in hormones or a condition you are already managing that just needs to be given special attention at this time.

Given how common mood disorders are during pregnancy and after childbirth, major obstetrical and midwifery organizations and the American Medical Association recommend that women be screened for mood disorders at least once during pregnancy. That doesn't mean, of course, that all providers (including yours) will do so, so it's important for you to understand this common complication of pregnancy and ask that your provider screen you for the conditions.

The good news is that, just like gestational diabetes, these conditions are very treatable, and there are concrete steps you can take to feel better if you experience one. You deserve to feel as strong as you can during pregnancy, so let's talk about this.

Factors That Put You at Risk for Developing a Mood Disorder in Pregnancy

- A history of anxiety or depression before pregnancy
- Experiencing medical complications during pregnancy
- Unplanned pregnancy
- Inadequate social support
- A history of trauma or abuse

For a full list of perinatal mood and anxiety disorders and the symptoms that can accompany them, see pages 205–227.

THE EFFECTS OF DEPRESSION IN PREGNANCY

Well, here's one of the biggest: you feel lousy during a time you hoped to enjoy. And that all by itself is reason enough to seek out experienced mental health care and take steps to feel better. But there are other reasons why you should prioritize your emotional health in pregnancy.

"Studies have shown that women who are depressed during pregnancy tend to have less compliance with prenatal care, they tend to have increased stress, which means they have more stress hormones flowing in their system and potentially crossing the placenta and reaching the baby—that's not such a great thing," says Howard. "Depressed pregnant moms may not be getting adequate sleep, eating well, or drinking enough liquids. They may also be more likely to self-medicate by smoking or using alcohol during pregnancy, and they are at increased risk for harming themselves."

Then there's the fact that "depression during pregnancy is one of the more robust predictors of postpartum depression," says Nonacs. All the more reason to get help early and start feeling better.

WHOM SHOULD I TALK TO?

If you feel comfortable with your obstetrician or midwife (and I hope you do; if not, switch!), be open with them about what you are feeling. He or she can refer you to a mental health provider, preferably one who specializes in reproductive mental health. You can also reach out to those providers directly (see page 370). No matter where you start talking, don't stop until someone commits to finding you help.

WILL I HAVE TO GO ON MEDICATION?

Not necessarily. There are several treatments available for anxiety and depression during pregnancy, including psychotherapy. In fact, says Vivien K. Burt, MD, codirector of the Women's Life Center at the Resnick Neuropsychiatric Hospital at UCLA, "for mild to moderate depression, psychotherapy works as well as medication." And Howard says that mild to moderate depression also responds well to a specific kind of therapy called cognitive behavioral therapy (CBT), in which you work on changing the way you think about certain situations as well as complementary modalities, such as prenatal yoga, acupuncture, and exercise. "All of these things have been shown to be beneficial," says Howard.

However, there are times when medication may be needed to return you to your normal functioning self, and it's important to know that if your provider determines that medication is the best treatment option for you, there are medications that experts are comfortable prescribing during pregnancy.

MAKING A DECISION ABOUT GOING ON MEDICATION

"Every month, there are new articles that come out about the risks and benefits of using or not using medications in pregnancies. None of the studies are perfect," says Burt. That's because randomized controlled studies are rarely conducted with pregnant women. So "when we talk to expectant mothers or women who would like to have a baby and face challenges such as anxiety, depression, panic disorder, or OCD," says Burt, "we say, 'Look, we can't guarantee everything or anything, but let's look at where you are, what we do know, and what you can comfortably live with.'"

Burt and her colleague Sonya Rasminsky wrote an article for *The Washington Post* entitled, "The 'Good Enough' Mother Begins in Pregnancy," in which they argue that striving for perfection in any area of motherhood is folly, especially when it comes to prioritizing your mental health.

Antidepressants may carry risks for obstetric outcomes and the health of offspring, but so do depression and anxiety themselves; there is no such thing as a risk-free decision; since no two expectant mothers (and their partners) are the same, the "right" or "best" decision for one couple is not the same as for another; and—this is important—the vast majority of babies do fine.

IF YOU ARE CURRENTLY ON MEDICATION FOR A MOOD OR ANXIETY DISORDER

It's important that before making any decisions about stopping or switching medications you speak with a health-care provider who has experience prescribing medication during pregnancy. While there are few gold-standard randomized trials of medications (of *all* sorts, not just psychiatric) on pregnant women, there is significant data, gathered after the fact, from women who were monitored during and after, that gives us information about the potential risks and benefits of any kind of medication during pregnancy.

"Many women get pregnant and their OB says, 'I don't know that medication,' and they come off it really abruptly," says Nonacs. And that can put both you and your baby at risk. In fact, untreated depression during pregnancy comes with its own risk factors.

Burt has studied what happens when women who are on medication for depression decide to discontinue during pregnancy. "Our study, published in *The Journal of the American Medical Association*, showed that the women who were kept on medication did well compared to those who stopped medication because they got pregnant." In fact, 75 percent of the women who stopped their medication became depressed again during pregnancy, compared to 25 percent of those women who chose to continue their treatment. "We know that medication can protect against a recurrence of depression," says Burt.

Psychotherapy as a Tool in Pregnancy and Motherhood

I began seeing a therapist halfway through my first pregnancy, when the anxiety of an unknown medical condition was mounting. Not only was she incredibly helpful with that specific issue, but she became my partner through all the ups and downs of pregnancy and new motherhood and was indispensable when I experienced postpartum anxiety. Without her, I would not have the understanding and calm and recovery to write this book and help other moms who feel like I did. (Thank you, DD.)

Sessions with a therapist can be the ultimate act of self-care during this time of your life. They offer you time to slow down and focus on yourself with someone trained in exactly what you are going through, whose whole job is to listen to—and support—you.

"If you've ever thought *maybe I should go to therapy*, pregnancy can be a wonderful time to do it," says Ariel Flavin, LCSW, a psychotherapist in Brooklyn (and one of my best friends). "Motherhood is a magnification of all that you are. All your struggles and all of your positives become magnified. So, why not make sure you know every crevice of yourself as much as you can beforehand? It can help you clarify and solidify who you are so that you will be able to see and hear yourself more clearly through all the fog and noise of parenthood. It's like spring cleaning before you add another person to your home."

See page 367 for how to find a therapist, including how to find low-cost care.

If you are currently taking medication for a mood disorder or considering starting one, find a psychiatrist or obstetric provider with experience prescribing medication during pregnancy. Look for a maternal fetal medicine expert or a reproductive psychiatrist (see page 370 for how to find one). Even if there is not one in your area, you can ask your provider to consult with one. There are also excellent, evidence-based online resources on medications in pregnancy that your provider can consult (see page 367). Once you have good information, you and your provider can discuss the pros and cons of continuing, starting, or switching medication.

The next step is putting in place a self-care plan that will reduce the stressors you experience during pregnancy, such as learning how to get good sleep (see page 64), trying yoga or other stress-relieving exercise (see page 72), and putting a plan in place to improve your emotional resilience after delivery (see page 134).

If You Have a History of Trauma

Women who have a history of trauma or abuse, particularly sexual abuse, are at increased risk for developing a mood or anxiety disorder during or after pregnancy.

"It is not uncommon for women who have had trauma earlier in their life to begin to re-experience traumatic memories, have nightmares, and feel more anxious during pregnancy," says Margaret Howard, PhD. That's in part, says Howard, because pregnancy, birth, and breastfeeding are unique physical experiences that can stir up emotions women thought they had worked through or suppressed.

"I've had patients who have a history of sexual abuse and are now living wonderful lives, have a baby, and come to me and say, 'I don't know what's happening. I'm crying all the time, I'm having nightmares—it's like I'm back in it again.' It's important that women who have trauma histories know this can happen; that way, they might feel less overwhelmed and more apt to recognize it and seek the treatment they need [see page 367]. These conditions are all treatable, but women should not wait."

Been There, Done That: Moms Share Stories of Mood and Anxiety Disorders During Pregnancy

---

I had a bout of depression. It was particularly bad in the second trimester, when everyone was telling me that I should be feeling great now that the nausea had passed. I found relief through weekly acupuncture sessions.

—Mom of a Toddler in North Carolina

I was quite anxious during my first pregnancy and managed it by going to therapy and doing quite a lot of journaling. I also found the book Birthing from Within *helpful for working through my emotions about pregnancy and birth.*   —Carrie, Saint Paul, Minnesota

I learned after a sixteen-week miscarriage in a prior pregnancy that I have a blood-clotting disorder that had caused my loss, and I was just terrified that it would happen again. I think some amount of that was just normal.

I suspect some amount was PTSD, and then I had some postpartum anxiety that led me to go on medication.

—Mom of One in Decatur, Georgia

I was diagnosed with bipolar disorder long before my pregnancy. I took precautions and had signed up to see a therapist at the hospital where I was delivering. If you already have any mental health problems, even in the past, or have a genetic predisposition, I would suggest doing the same thing if you possibly can. A therapist hopefully can catch if you are going from tired new mom to a serious problem.

—Nicole, West Virginia

I had very mild anxiety before pregnancy. I'd been on Prozac and stopped. I decided not to get back on it after the baby, which was a mistake. With number two, I went home with a prescription.

—Meredith, Decatur, Georgia

I was told by my general practitioner—when I mentioned that I wanted to get pregnant—that I was going to have to wean off my depression medication. My whole pregnancy I was depressed and the first six months after, because nobody would let me go on medication when I was breastfeeding. It was really awful, but now I know that it doesn't have to be awful. I thought I was being a good mother, but I could have been a better mom if I hadn't stopped medication for my sanity that was potentially bad for my baby's "health."

—Jane, Los Angeles, California

Making Self-Care Second Nature

The second trimester is usually seen as the pregnancy sweet spot. The time when the nausea, vomiting, and exhaustion of the first hopefully let up, your energy may pick up, sex just might seem appealing again, and you will undoubtedly begin to show.

For many, these changes are positive and welcome and signal a settling into your pregnancy. For others, the nausea may continue, energy may still be hard to find, and showing might bring new emotions that are not what you expected. Just like in the first trimester, allowing yourself to feel whatever emotions come up for you and taking care of yourself should be your two big priorities. In fact, the comparative calm of the second trimester offers you an opportunity to kick self-care into gear and really plan for how you will take care of yourself during the third trimester and when you are a new mom.

So this section is loaded with tips on getting comfortable in your growing body, managing nosy questions from strangers and setting boundaries, practical tips for actually getting sleep, and some seriously useful advice for sex that will take you all the way into new parenthood.

FIND OUT WHAT MAKES YOU HAPPY

If you think about it, you can probably quickly come up with activities you enjoy, ones that help you feel calm, give you energy, or feel like an escape. What are they? Make a list of times in your life when you felt centered and think back to what you were doing then.

Whatever your particular pursuits—walking, running, reading books, having lunch with good friends, writing in your journal in a coffee shop, making art, or just having some alone time in any form—make a list and begin to work these activities into your daily or weekly routine. Just like exercising a muscle or rehearsing a musical instrument, your ability to take care of yourself will strengthen the more you practice it. If you make time to yourself a nonnegotiable now, you are much more likely to stick with it after pregnancy.

"I think that a lot of parenting books and mainstream culture give parents this idea that our child is our primary activity and we need to fit our self-care into the nooks and crannies that are left over after we've met our child's needs," says Carla Naumburg, PhD, author of *Parenting in the Present Moment: How to Stay Focused on What Really Matters*. "But assuming a parent is taking care of their child's basic needs, then from there they can figure out how to fit their kid into *their* needs."

And all that takes is modifying your routine so that your child can fit into it. For instance, if Zumba is your jam, then find a YMCA or gym that offers childcare while you shimmy your stress away. If you love to run or walk, put a top-quality baby jogger on your registry. If you're an artist or just love to make crafts, put a bouncy seat on your registry, treat yourself to some good supplies, and have them ready to bring out in moments when your little one is happily bouncing away. Or see if that YMCA offers art classes for adults.

The more central and baby-friendly you make self-care, the harder it will be to push aside when you are a mom.

Feeling Good About Your Changing Body

Probably not since puberty has your body been through such a massive change, one that feels emotionally volatile but also alters how you look on the outside. Some women feel empowered by their bodies' ability to grow a human being. Others may feel an alien being has taken over their bodies. And with all the pressure women face in our society to have a certain type of body, being pregnant can dredge up body-image issues simmering beneath the surface.

"All the emphasis on how pregnant women look leads to an underlying anxiety of 'I hope this happens the right way,'" says Jodi Rubin, LCSW, an eating disorder specialist in Manhattan, who works with pregnant women. "The reality is that there is no right way. Everybody's different."

If women are having difficulty adjusting to their changing bodies, Rubin suggests reframing the way they are thinking about them. "If you can, move the focus from how different your body feels and, instead, take time to acknowledge the beauty in it, that it is creating a life." But she also acknowledges that there are people who just don't like being pregnant. "I try not to approach pregnancy with the assumption that everybody's going to love it," says Rubin.

She also recommends ignoring the unrealistic portrayals of celebrity pregnancies. "This is not what people look like," says Rubin. Instead, connect with real women online or in person who are working through the *real* changes of pregnancy so you can share your concerns and feel less alone.

Rubin also tells women who are struggling with body-image issues to ask their providers not to tell them their weight each visit. "There is no reason for anyone to know their weight during pregnancy," says Rubin. "Your practitioner is the only one who needs that information."

WHAT IF I AM WORRYING TOO MUCH ABOUT MY WEIGHT?

The natural anxiety around pregnancy and the added focus on weight can be a trigger for women who have experienced eating disorders or can introduce a distorted relationship with their bodies and food.

So if your concerns about your body image and food choices start to cause you anxiety or occupy your thoughts much of the time, it might be a good idea to touch base with a mental health professional who specializes in body image (see page 365).

Whether you have had an eating disorder in the past or not, the following red flags are signs that you should definitely find some professional support to help you feel better and take good care of yourself:

- Restricting food or eating low-fat and low-calorie meals with the intention of avoiding weight gain
- Skipping meals (maybe before a weigh-in at the doctor's office)
- Your exercise routine is causing you discomfort, but you won't modify it
- You are having persistent intrusive thoughts about your body and anxiety about it
- You are bingeing or purging

Even if you aren't experiencing any of these behaviors but you have a history of an eating disorder and you feel worried about your body changing so much, Rubin says it's worth talking to a professional.

Been There, Done That: Moms Share How They Felt About Their Bodies

---

I felt love and appreciation for my body in a new way.
—KIMBERLY, WASHINGTON, DC

I remember feeling disappointed that people didn't realize I was pregnant until pretty late in my pregnancy and therefore must've just thought that I was fat. But I also remember feeling devastated the first time a stranger realized that I was pregnant. My husband didn't understand how I could possibly be upset by both people not *recognizing that I was pregnant and by people who* did *realize I was pregnant.*
—EMILY T.

I felt super attractive, strong, and beautiful.

—Carrie, Saint Paul, Minnesota.

I loved my pregnant body. For probably the only time in my life, my "shape" was totally acceptable for what it was, needed no explanation, and carried no guilt.

—Kendra, Atlanta, Georgia

I loved having boobs.   —Jen, Portland, Oregon

"You're Huge!" and Other Things
People Say and Do

- "Oh, wow! Are you having twins?"
- "Oh my gosh. You're so little, I didn't even realize you were pregnant."
- "Better get your sleep now. It's your last chance!"
- "You're not going to get the epidural, right?"
- "Are you going to have a 'natural' birth?"
- "I didn't think it was okay to eat deli meat during pregnancy."
- "Looks like you won't have any trouble breastfeeding!"
- "You're about to pop!"

Once you start to show, the world knows you're pregnant and the world wants to talk about it. A lot. It's like the fact that another person is growing inside you gives every person on the planet permission to say anything and everything that comes into their head. Or to even reach out and touch your belly, something they would never think to do if you were not pregnant.

I recognize that many of these interactions come from a good place. There *is* something really magical—unbelievable,

he ability to grow a human being inside you, but
don't know what to do with their fascination or
t with you. So you end up hearing a lot of re-
, comments, and questions that can either feel
like really fun attention, drive you nuts, or, in some cases,
make you anxious.

GETTING SIZED UP

If you are concerned about your weight gain in pregnancy,
comments on your size can send you to Google for two hours
researching gestational diabetes. For women who carry small,
hearing comments like "You don't even look pregnant!" can
launch a host of worries in their heads about the baby's development. "A lot about pregnancy is unpredictable," says Kathryn L. Bleiberg, PhD, associate professor of psychology in
clinical psychiatry at Weill Cornell Medicine in New York
City, "but one thing you can predict is that people are going
to comment on how you are carrying, and some of those comments you won't like."

Understanding that this is a common experience for all
women who are pregnant will make the comments feel less
personal. It's also important to remember that the man in line
at the grocery store or the woman at the gas station are not
medical experts. Women carry in many different ways, and
"only you and your OB know about your body and pregnancy,"
says Bleiberg. So talk to him or her if you are concerned. As for
that annoying comment on the bus? "You can address it, or you
can change the subject," says Rubin. "Just say, 'Thank you, I
feel really good,' and move on. You don't have to have the conversation."

GETTING FELT UP

I'm pretty sure that there is some kind of invisible magnet inside a pregnant woman's belly that attracts the hands of certain people. I get it. I have this urge anytime I am near a good friend who is pregnant, and I have to consciously tell myself not to act on the urge or to ask first. Not everyone is similarly restrained.

It's totally understandable if touch from friends or strangers is uncomfortable to you, and it's 100 percent okay for you to step away, ask people not to, or let them know it makes you feel uncomfortable. In fact, I wrote an article on the topic and my favorite comeback came from pregnancy etiquette expert Paula Spencer Scott, author of *Momfidence!: An Oreo Never Killed Anybody and Other Secrets of Happier Parenting.* "Just tell them, 'Look, but don't touch!' or 'You break it, you buy it.'" Humor is an easy way to set a boundary, but it's also perfectly acceptable to be straightforward. "Tell them that it feels uncomfortable. You don't have to be specific about whether it's an emotional or physical response," advises Scott.

GETTING UNSOLICITED ADVICE AND NOSY QUESTIONS

Many (all?) pregnancy and parenting choices are personal, and some you can't prepare for until you face them, but that won't stop people you barely know from asking if you plan to get an epidural, whether you want to breastfeed, and who will be staying home to take care of the baby. And these kinds of inquiries are usually served up with a healthy side of unsolicited advice.

· ·
Good Pregnancy Comebacks and Distracting Techniques
· ·

- "Everybody carries differently. I'm feeling great."
- "Growing a person inside of you is kind of amazing, right?"
- "Thanks, but I don't really like talking about my body. Can we talk about something else?"
- "Thanks. I feel really strong. How are you doing?"
- "I know! Isn't pregnancy crazy?"
- "Oh, great, another thing to worry about!"
- "We haven't decided yet."
- "How did you make a decision about that?"
- "That's really a private matter between my partner and me."
- "Hands off the merchandise!"
- "What was your favorite thing about being pregnant?"
- "What was the hardest?"
- "Would you excuse me? I have to go to the bathroom."

HEARING WORST-CASE SCENARIOS

No scientific data on this one, but it's safe to say that many people like to talk about themselves and their experiences. Put that together with the fact that the best stories usually involve conflict and drama, and you end up with people sharing their pregnancy, birth, and parenthood horror stories with you. I really don't think people think it through before they share intimate details of the hemorrhoids they had after vaginal birth or give you the blow by blow of their sister's emergency C-section, or drop a bomb like, "Sleep as much as you can now. I haven't slept through the night in three years."

Maybe they want to feel less alone in the experiences they went through, or maybe they want to share information with you they wish they had had. Whatever the motivation, these comments are all about the person sharing them and have no factual bearing on your pregnancy, and you are under no obligation to listen to them.

PRACTICE SETTING BOUNDARIES NOW

Pregnancy is a great time to practice putting boundaries in place. When you become a mom, you are embarking on an endeavor that other people feel they have a stake in—whether they are close family members who are related to your child or random members of society who believe they have a say in how future citizens are raised. The fact is that you will be hearing a lot of opinions from a lot of people from here on out.

Take this time to explore your thoughts, feelings, beliefs, plans, and hopes for parenthood (this book should help you with a lot of that), to get comfortable *not* knowing exactly how you will act in a given situation, and to practice standing up for what matters to you and letting people know when you do or do *not* want their input. "*No* can be a really loving word," says Christina Hibbert, PsyD, a clinical psychologist in Flagstaff, Arizona, who specializes in women's mental health and motherhood, "because you are saying yes to something better—the fact that you are the authority on you and your family."

Been There, Done That: Moms Share Stories of How
They Handled Pregnancy Comments and Nosy Questions

---

*When people would touch my belly, I reached out and did
the same to them. It freaked people out and made me feel sort
of empowered.* —LAUREL, ATLANTA, GEORGIA

*Something that bothered me were the "You need to do this"
comments. "You need to breastfeed." "You need to let them
sleep in a crib by X months." I felt like, "This is my baby and
my personal experience. Feel free to give me suggestions and
advice, but please don't tell me what I have to or absolutely
cannot do."* —DOMINGA, SAINT PAUL, MINNESOTA

*People were very nice. I had more doors opened and more
people offer to help and carry things for me. I enjoyed it.*
—STEPHANIE, DALLAS, TEXAS

*There are so many annoying things people say to pregnant
solo moms. So many assumptions and projections of what
your story is—either on your side (when you don't necessarily
need it) because they have a divorced sister or, weirdly, on
the father's side (without knowing him) because they have a
divorced brother with a difficult ex-wife. And the dreaded
"Who's the father?" question that no one asks a married
woman even if they have never met her partner. Separate
your truth and reality from their often well-meaning projections and assumptions.*
—DOMENICA, BROOKLYN, NEW YORK

*When I was eight-and-a-half-months pregnant, I went to
get a pedicure and foot massage. Right in the middle—when
I was feeling so happy and relaxed—a woman walked into
the salon and said very loudly, "How can you expose your
unborn child to all of those fumes? Shame on you!" and
walked out. I was so taken by surprise that I didn't say anything. I sat there suddenly feeling guilty and judged and the
opposite of relaxed. For weeks, I fantasized about what I
wished I would have said to her. I have tried so hard ever
since to never make another mother feel judged.*

—Jen, Portland, Oregon

Why Sleep Matters and How to Get It

Research shows that getting good sleep is one of the most important things we can do for our physical and mental health. It is as important as eating and breathing. Sleep helps our bodies and brains repair themselves, helps us consolidate memories and process information, and be able to focus. And *not* getting good sleep has been shown to increase the risk of mood disorders and lead to irritability and loss of concentration, among many other things.

"Sleep is the foundation for everything," says author and parenting coach Carla Naumburg, PhD. "Trying to function well when we are exhausted is a little bit like trying to drive a car with a flat tire." Which is why learning how to get good sleep should be at the very top of your pregnancy and parenting priorities.

"SAY GOODBYE TO A GOOD NIGHT'S SLEEP!"

The idea that you will sleep poorly in pregnancy (and then in parenthood) is so widely accepted that almost nothing is done to help women get good sleep when they are pregnant or new parents. In fact, 60 percent of women experience insomnia during pregnancy and early parenthood compared with only 12 percent of women who are not pregnant or new parents.

"I get the sense that a lot of OBs perceive sleep deprivation in pregnancy as normal," says Leslie Swanson, PhD, a sleep specialist and clinical assistant professor at the University of Michigan. And the rest of us buy into the expectation that you just won't get good sleep until your kid goes to college. "We tend to minimize the effects of sleep disruption or insomnia during the perinatal period," says Swanson. "We assume it's normal."

Learning how to get good sleep is not only going to help you feel much better during pregnancy, it is also going to be a critical skill on your parenthood journey. "Women who have poor sleep have more symptoms of anxiety and depression or are at greater risk for developing depression," says Swanson. "Poor sleep late in pregnancy is also tied to an increased chance of depression after delivery," says Swanson.

WHY IT'S HARD TO SLEEP DURING PREGNANCY

More than half of pregnant women experience insomnia, and that's because pregnancy creates "the perfect storm for it," says Swanson. Start with the fact that you are female—a major risk factor for insomnia (in fact, a recent study found that 12.8 percent of women experienced insomnia compared with 9.7 percent of men). Then add the fact that life changes increase your risk (Hello! Pregnancy!). And finally, hormones can wreak havoc with circadian rhythms (your biological clock, which tells you when to be awake and when to sleep). Combine all that with the physical discomfort of pregnancy, and it's easy to see why a good night's sleep can begin to feel like a mythical aspiration.

"In early pregnancy, probably the biggest impact on sleep is hormonal," says Katherine M. Sharkey, MD, PhD, associate professor of medicine and psychiatry and human behavior at Brown University. "There are massive increases in progesterone, which act on the same receptor system that most sleeping pills act on. So a lot of women will say how exhausted they feel during that first trimester. As pregnancy progresses, sleep is interrupted by a whole range of things, from more physical symptoms, having to go to the bathroom frequently, acid reflux, and worrying."

How to Get Better Sleep

Things Anyone Can Do

- No caffeine in the afternoon
- No computer or phone use an hour before bed (the blue light emitted from electronic devices disrupts your body's production of the sleep hormone melatonin)
- Reserve your bed for sleep and sex only
- Make your bedtime and wake time consistent to strengthen your circadian rhythm
- Keep your bedroom cool, quiet, and dark
- Read relaxing material (no murder mysteries or intense magazine articles!) before bed
- Try relaxation techniques or meditation apps, such as Headspace

- Use calming aromatherapy scents, like lavender, in the bedroom

What Pregnant Women Can Add to That List

- Use extra pillows to support your belly as it grows (see "Been There, Done That")
- Reduce your fluid intake before bed, so the need to pee doesn't wake you
- If you have heartburn, don't eat less than four hours before bed, elevate the head of your bed with pillows or elements added under the mattress or frame, try taking TUMS, and ask your doctor about medication to reduce heartburn
- If you find your mind running through all the baby preparation to-dos, keep a list by your bed so you can download your brain before bed or quickly write things down in the middle of the night and return to sleep
- Set aside a "worry time" a few hours before bed; sit down and think about the things that are weighing on your mind; jot down notes or to-dos if you want, and then let yourself focus on other thoughts once you are in bed

WHAT IF I STILL CAN'T SLEEP?

"It is crucial that you get your sleep problems addressed and identified by someone who will treat you for it," advises Swanson. Typically, doctors diagnose insomnia when a person experiences one of three things—trouble falling asleep, trouble staying asleep, or waking too early—for three or more nights a week for at least three months. But pregnant women don't have three months to see if their sleep is a problem. "If a pregnant woman considers it a problem, we want to address it," says Swanson, "because we know that when a woman considers her sleep problematic is when the increased risk for depression comes into play."

The medications used to treat sleep disorders, such as zolpidem (Ambien), have not been well studied in pregnancy, although some obstetricians will opt for medications such as Benadryl, which have been used widely during pregnancy and can help you sleep. But perhaps the most effective treatment for insomnia—cognitive behavioral therapy—involves no medication. A sleep specialist works with you to pinpoint what in your habits, routine, or home may be contributing to your sleep difficulty and creates a targeted plan to make changes in those areas.

Common Sleep Disorders in Pregnancy

Restless leg syndrome affects as many as one in four pregnant women. Women experience uncomfortable sensations in their arms and/or legs. The symptoms usually hit in the late afternoon or early evening and give women the urge to move their legs to relieve discomfort. Some people say it feels like pins and needles or like someone is touching them. One of the most effective treatments for RLS is iron, which can be safely supplemented in pregnancy under the care of an expert, says Katherine M. Sharkey, MD. "Other medications may also be warranted in certain situations."

Sleep Disordered Breathing Refers to a Range of Disorders—from Snoring to Obstructive Sleep Apnea

These conditions are more common during pregnancy for a couple of reasons, including weight gain, increased swelling in the tissues around your throat, and pressure on the diaphragm from your uterus. Though snoring may seem more like an annoyance than a health issue, it's actually a symptom of a medical problem that should be evaluated by a medical professional. These conditions can be treated safely during pregnancy with a continuous positive airway pressure (CPAP) machine. You wear a mask over your nose and mouth and the machine blows air through your nose to keep your throat from closing off.

PRACTICING PARENTHOOD SLEEP

Kathryn Lee, RN, professor emerita at the University of California at San Francisco School of Nursing, is a sleep specialist who has devoted her career to helping expectant and new moms get some z's, and her research has uncovered some useful information. In one of her studies, she created some of the conditions moms would experience in the newborn period so that women could practice during pregnancy.

Using only first-time moms, Lee randomly gave half of them a bedside bassinet, a nightlight, and a sound machine. She instructed them to put the nightlight and sound machine on a power strip under the bassinet to allow a little light so moms would be able to feed and diaper their babies safely during night wakings. The sound machine was to help mask the little noises babies make—gurgling, heavy breathing—

but wouldn't mask the louder cries of hunger or distress. Members of the control group in the study were given educational information about sleep hygiene and the effects of alcohol and caffeine on sleep.

She found that the changes in the bedroom environment to prepare for infant care during the night were effective in getting more sleep in the newborn period. At one month and at three months after birth, the moms who practiced for the newborn period were getting thirty minutes more sleep a night.

Been There, Done That: Moms Talk About Getting Sleep (or Not) During Pregnancy

---

Pillows! Pillows! Pillows! Literally between every joint.
— ALI, PHILADELPHIA, PENNSYLVANIA

Beginning in the second trimester, sleep was more difficult. I adjusted my sleep schedule. I went to bed earlier, because I knew I could fall asleep quickly, but I would often wake up around 4:00 A.M. and was unable to fall back asleep. I would lie in bed until 5:00, and if I was still awake by then, I'd get up for the day.
— ELIZABETH, SAINT PAUL, MINNESOTA

Chamomile tea.   — LIZ, LONDON, UK

Between getting up to pee, getting comfortable, getting leg cramps, and getting heartburn, it was pretty difficult. I found that one of the only things that helped near the end of my pregnancy was TUMS with calcium and potassium. They helped the leg cramps as well!   —EMILY

Sleeping was awful! I'd had sleep apnea for years, but it was mild and manageable. Once I got to about the six-month mark, I couldn't sleep at all. Finally, around eight months I got a CPAP, and that was a godsend.

—RACHEL, CANBERRA, AUSTRALIA

I started up a relationship with my body pillow, Ed, during my first pregnancy, and I kept him around through the second. He still sleeps at the head of our bed for when I need him. He's so good that I once packed Ed in his own suitcase and checked him onto a plane.

—JEN, PORTLAND, OREGON

Moving Your Body Will Improve Your Mood

Like sleep, exercise is one of those "luxuries" that are often the first to go in times of stress. But exercise is also like sleep in that it is one of the most important things you can prioritize to help manage your mood and build the strength to weather all the new stresses in your life.

Of course, pregnancy can seem like a wonderful excuse to take a break from your fitness routine (or to delay starting one)—and some conditions in, or complications of, pregnancy necessitate slowing way down or stopping altogether (that's a conversation for you and your health-care provider). But for those who are able, keeping your body moving will not only help regulate your mood in pregnancy, it will make it much easier to keep doing it when it matters most and is hardest to do—the first three months postpartum.

During my first pregnancy, I ran three times a week until Braxton Hicks contractions in the second trimester made it too uncomfortable. Then I walked for a while. Then I stopped. In my second pregnancy, I went to my favorite spin class once a week (and I loved it), but otherwise I was fairly sedentary (well, as sedentary as you can be when you live in New York City without a car). So I come to this section with no judgment, but I also arrive here as a parent who did not have a regular fitness routine until her first child was eight years old. Now that I do, I see the incredible impact it has on my happiness, mental fitness, energy, and confidence, and I wish I had known this back when I was pregnant with my first kid.

But don't take it from me! Listen to the experts. First up: the American Congress of Obstetricians and Gynecologists (ACOG), which recommends thirty minutes of exercise most days of the week for women who do not have a health condition or pregnancy complication that would prevent them from exercising. (Oh, and here is where I have to add one of those legal disclaimers about how you should absolutely talk to your health-care provider before beginning or continuing a vigorous exercise routine in pregnancy. And, that's true, you should.)

HOW EXERCISE IMPACTS YOUR EVERYDAY MOOD

"Exercise not only releases endorphins (feel-good chemicals) but has been shown to actually increase the neurotransmitter levels in our brain just like antidepressants do," says psychologist Christina Hibbert, PsyD. In addition, exercise can improve your mood, because it improves your energy and "bad moods are really an energy issue," says Hibbert. Plus, exercise is a proven stress reducer—and pregnancy is actually viewed in the world of psychology as a stressor, according to Melanie Poudevigne, PhD, director of health and fitness management at Clayton State University in Morrow, Georgia. There is, unfortunately, limited research on exercise in pregnancy, but "what we do know is that in pregnant women, inactivity worsens mood," says Poudevigne.

HOW EXERCISE CAN HELP WITH MOOD AND ANXIETY DISORDERS

"There is a lot of research that shows the benefit of exercise in reducing fear and worry as well as the symptoms of depression, anxiety, and a variety of mental illnesses like bipolar disorder," says Hibbert. In fact, one major study found that people with major depressive disorder who exercised for a half hour three to five times per week reduced their symptoms of depression by nearly 50 percent.

"Most forms of exercise will improve mood disorders," says Poudevigne. "The physical exercise will improve your serotonin level [the same thing antidepressants do], and that will improve your symptoms." In order to see this benefit, Poudevigne says you need to exercise at moderate intensity for twenty minutes three to five days of the week.

EXERCISE IS NOT A SUBSTITUTE FOR MEDICAL TREATMENT IF YOU NEED IT

"Exercise is a wonderful option for mild to moderate depression or when someone is emerging from depression," says psychiatrist Vivien K. Burt, MD. "But if someone is feeling paralyzed from depression, exercise is not a replacement for treatment. In fact, being told to exercise can make you feel worse about yourself. It's like somebody telling somebody who is anxious to 'just relax.'" For more information on depression and other mood disorders during pregnancy, see pages 38–47.

. . . .
Ways to Make Exercise a Routine
. . . .

- **Keep a notebook by the door** and write down how you feel before you move your body and then after. Pretty quickly it should be clear the mood boost you are getting from exercise.
- **Walk in the morning before work** or during your lunch break; don't leave it until you get home and the rush of the evening or your exhaustion gets the better of you.
- **Make regular plans to exercise with friends.** Accountability is one of the most effective things you can do to stick to an exercise routine.
- **Try prenatal yoga or Pilates classes.** YMCAs, community centers, and city public health departments offer free or low-cost options.
- **Let go of all-or-nothing thinking.** Gradually work up to the recommended amount.
- **Put a fitness tracker on your registry** and ask someone to give it to you early. You can set a daily goal for steps as well as the number of minutes you are active.
- **Know that the first twenty minutes are the hardest** and then it gets easier.
- **Remember that exercise is not a selfish pursuit** but a seriously effective way to improve your mood (and physical health!) and allow you to return to your family refreshed.

· ·

Basic Safety Tips for Exercising in Pregnancy

· ·

- **Talk to your health-care provider** before starting any exercise routine or continuing any strenuous routine.

- **Monitor your intensity.** You should be able to talk, but it should be a little difficult. If you can chat away, you are not exercising enough. If you can't talk, it's too much.

- **Hydrate often.** Check that your urine is light yellow and not dark to ensure you are staying hydrated.

- **Wear loose clothing** that will allow your sweat to evaporate.

- **Do not exercise when you are hungry.**

- **Exercise in cool indoor spaces** during hot weather.

- **Stop doing any exercises lying on your back** after your fourth month.

- **Avoid contact sports** and activities that could easily lead to injury, such as horseback riding or downhill skiing.

Been There, Done That: Moms Talk About Exercising During Pregnancy

---

I walked and swam throughout. It was helpful for the anxiety and to keep my strength up for the delivery.

—DIANE, HUDSON VALLEY, NEW YORK

I had gestational diabetes, so I exercised to get my glucose numbers in range. It gave me needed energy, kept my head clear. —KENDRA, ATLANTA, GEORGIA

I did nothing with the first pregnancy. I felt like a giant blob. The second time, I exercised a lot up until about seven months. I felt great! —MEREDITH, DECATUR, GEORGIA

Pregnancy water aerobics was the best, because I felt so weightless! —BRIDGETTE

Yoga helped immensely. Also taking walks. I would increase the frequency of both of these if I could do it again. —ANONYMOUS

Sex During Pregnancy

Let's be honest about whether you do or don't want sex, and let's brainstorm ways to be intimate that will work for you and your partner. Some women find that the hormones of pregnancy "light a fire under their libido and they want more sex than before," says Erin Martinez, LMSW, a certified sex therapist in Dearborn, Michigan. For others, nausea, exhaustion, or other changes steal away any desire they have.

There are a million ways you might feel about sex right now. So here are some answers to questions you might have, some suggestions for having sex while pregnant, for staying intimate without sex, and for managing any discrepancy in the way you are feeling with how your partner is feeling. It's all about figuring out what feels comfortable to you and making that happen.

IS IT OKAY TO HAVE VAGINAL SEX WHEN YOU'RE PREGNANT?

This one is covered in most of the pregnancy books on your nightstand. And the expert answer is: as long as your health-care provider has not told you there is a reason that you cannot have sex, you are free to go for it. (Note: I am not a health-care provider.)

DOES THE BABY FEEL IT?

"A lot of people say they are worried sex will interfere with the baby or they don't think it's appropriate," says Martinez, but "research repeatedly shows that sexual intercourse does not hurt the baby. Your baby may know *something* is going on, but your baby does not know *what* is going on. Sperm can stimulate the uterus and "cause a tightening feeling, but that doesn't mean your baby is hurt," says Martinez.

WHAT IF I DON'T WANT TO?

There could be lots of reasons why sex during pregnancy does not appeal. "If you have morning sickness, smells, food, everything may turn you off," says Sarah Watson, LPC, a certified sex therapist in Rochester Hills, Michigan. "You may not want your partner to touch you." Even if you don't feel nauseous at every turn, you may just be taking some time to adjust to your news and your new body, and physical intimacy with someone else may not take priority right now.

But it is still nice to feel cared for and to have your presence desired. If you feel so terrible that touch is out of the question, explain that to your partner and try doing things that keep you close without requiring touch—like reading to each other from your favorite magazines or a good book.

If being touched does feel nice, ask for back rubs, cuddle together on the couch while you binge-watch your favorite

TV show, fall asleep holding hands, or just spend some time in bed feeling the baby move and looking into each other's eyes. There's a little life growing inside you. That can be a pretty intimate moment to savor.

WHAT IF MY PARTNER DOES BUT I DON'T?

"Be really honest," says Watson. "I think most women have a difficult time communicating about our bodies—pregnant or not—so let this moment give you the power to say what you are feeling." Doing so will set the stage for open conversations throughout your pregnancy and into parenthood. "An easy way to start is just to express how you are feeling (rather than starting with what you see your partner doing or not doing), like, "I need to talk with you about what's been going on with me."

WHAT IF MY PARTNER DOESN'T WANT SEX?

If you feel your partner's interest in sex waning, ask him or her about whether it is. Some conversation starters: "How do you feel about my body now that I am pregnant?" "What parts are attractive to you now?" "Are you worried about anything?" "Are there other things we could do that you would enjoy?"

Whatever you are feeling, the important thing is to maintain your connection and open up a conversation about sex so that you can talk about it as your pregnancy progresses. You may find you feel really differently depending on the trimester.

BUT MY VULVA LOOKS WEIRD AND
MY BREASTS HURT!

The changes of pregnancy can take some adjustment and exploration. (Don't get me started on the time three days of bed rest in my second trimester led to the Attack of the Giant Labia. Let's just say it's not a great moment when your partner has to be on the phone with your OB while scrutinizing the state of your vulva and describing what your labia look like to see if it's a concern.)

But enough about my awesome labia; take the nipples and breasts (no, don't; I need them!). How they feel differs for different women. Sensitivity may increase, making them a more enjoyable part of physical intimacy, or they may feel too tender, and, toward the end of pregnancy, engorged and full of feeding purpose. Maybe you don't want your partner anywhere near them. Your vulva is also likely a little bigger and a little darker with the increased blood flow down there (hopefully not as big as mine got; sorry, I'm talking about my labia again). This might make you uncomfortable with something like oral sex, or it may increase your sensitivity and feel great. Explore these areas and find out what feels good and what doesn't and then tell each other.

WHAT CAN I DO INSTEAD OF SEX?

So much! "Any straight guy with gay friends eventually confides that he's jealous that they have so much more sex than he does," says Dan Savage, author of the long-running sex advice column Savage Love and creator of the *Savage Lovecast*.

"That's because we define a lot more things as sex. For straight people, sex is defined as vaginal intercourse, and anything else is a consolation prize."

"Sex and pregnancy is a great time to get away from the idea that intercourse is the only thing you do," agrees Martinez. "It opens up this huge spectrum of what might be enjoyable, exciting, close, and pleasurable." And this redefining of sex will really pay off in the postpartum period when penetration may be the last thing on your mind for weeks, months, or longer. Expanding your sex repertoire in pregnancy is a great way to set the stage for a return to intimacy after birth.

Savage recommends straight couples take a cue from their gay counterparts. "Every single gay encounter starts with the question: 'What are you into?' You can rule anything in or anything out. That's something heterosexual couples should steal—along with brunch and sit-ups."

Fun Ways to Expand Your Sexual Repertoire
- Hand jobs (for both of you)
- Oral sex
- Mutual masturbation
- Assisted masturbation (your partner holding you and maybe talking to you while you masturbate; you holding your partner and talking while he or she masturbates)
- Using toys
- Sharing fantasies and stories (could be sharing past sexual encounters or idealized encounters)
- Reading erotica to each other
- Making out on the couch

- Showering together and washing each other
- Taking a bath together if you have a big tub
- Naked touch like tickling, pinching, kissing with no specific end goal
- That other thing that just popped into your mind

If nothing else, spending time together relaxing physically can end in a great night's sleep—and in pregnancy, that *is* a happy ending.

Been There, Done That: Moms Share Stories of Sex in Pregnancy

It took us about four weeks to have sex for the first time, because my husband was anxious about harming me or the baby. We finally broke that anxiety through talk—and wine and Googling for him.

—Elizabeth, Saint Paul, Minnesota

We both enjoyed it a lot. I felt very sexy with curves and boobs and very intimate with a baby inside.

—Rachel, London, UK

Sex was stressful for me, because we had had several pregnancy losses. I knew rationally that having sex wouldn't harm the fetus, but that fear lingered. My husband and I talked about our different feelings. I respected that he wished we were more sexual, and he understood why I might be more reluctant, both physically and emotionally.

—Diana, Montclair, New Jersey

I was sad that my partner wasn't terribly into it. I think she was freaked out that we would hurt the baby.

—A Mom in Decatur, Georgia

I had a big sex drive, but hubby wouldn't initiate, and if I did, he would barely get into it. I took matters into my own hands most nights.

—Mom to a Toddler in the Carolinas

Once I was huge, I preferred to keep my shirt on because it took me out of the "sexy headspace" I was trying to maintain.   —Jo, Atlanta, Georgia

I had an "incompetent cervix," so I had stitches put in my cervix at twelve weeks. For seven months, we could not have vaginal intercourse. It was hard. I was scared he'd want to go somewhere else, even though I knew he never would. There were tears and lots of need for reassurance. He handled it all great and even went through it all again willingly with our second child. We also found other ways to have fun sexually.

—Dominga, Saint Paul, Minnesota

Managing the Emotions
of Pregnancy Complications
or a "High-Risk" Pregnancy

When I was pregnant with my first daughter, I developed a relatively benign but very painful and scary medical condition called *pericarditis*. The sac around my heart would get swollen at different times throughout the pregnancy (it always sounded like a country song to me: "My heart sac's swollen, and it hurts so bad!"). It's not a typical pregnancy complication (so don't start Googling it and worrying that you might have it). In my case, I had pericarditis a year before pregnancy, probably from a virus, and 30 percent of people who have one episode go on to have recurrent episodes. I was one of the unlucky third, and it seemed pregnancy was the trigger for recurrence.

Because it is not a typical complication, it went undiagnosed for half my pregnancy, landing me in the ER twice and the hospital, necessitating CT scans and nuclear medicine scans and other things you are told to avoid in pregnancy. After five months of uncertainty and fear, it was finally diagnosed. The treatment was ibuprofen, which I took sporadically in the second trimester. By the third trimester, ibuprofen couldn't control the inflammation, and I had to take steroids. Throughout that time, I was reading pregnancy books that suggested the safest approach to treating a headache was to just look at a Tylenol but not actually take one. And here I was pounding steroids like a bodybuilder.

One moment from that time that is seared into my memory is the sunlight-infused prenatal yoga class I went to the day I was released from a hospital stay. The teacher asked us to go around the room and say what our intention was for practice that day. Every other student talked about wanting to feel connected to her developing baby or prepare her body for "natural" birth. Here's what I said: "I just got out of the hospital, so I want to get back in touch with the idea that my body is strong and my baby will be born healthy." I felt like a freak. I was mad at—and jealous of—the other women. After the class, I cried.

That moment was one of several that made me want to write a book that represented *all* the experiences of pregnancy so that anyone who was struggling with something could find words in the pages that spoke to them and made them feel less alone. This section is about doing that for medical complications in pregnancy.

Whether you entered pregnancy with a preexisting condition that must be managed to ensure your health as well as the health of your baby or you developed complications as a result of pregnancy, you are not alone. But that doesn't mean it isn't really hard.

MAKING A HUMAN BEING IS HARD, COMPLICATED WORK

"Making a person on the planet Earth is really hard, and there's so much pressure to do things well. So have some self-compassion," says psychotherapist Sarah Best. "It's okay to say to yourself, 'It sucks that I have to deal with this.' No one wants to hear this, but the idea that pregnancy is supposed to be easy is just an idea. It may be that easy pregnancies are the exception and not the rule."

Totally Normal Feelings You May Be Having
- Anger (sometimes at the baby)
- Guilt over the anger or over not being as healthy as you had hoped to be
- Resentment
- Sadness at the loss of a worry-free pregnancy
- Jealousy of women who are having pregnancies without complications
- Feelings of being robbed of an experience you wanted and expected
- Anxiety
- Fear for your health or the health of your baby
- A sense of being out of control

LET YOURSELF FEEL THEM WITHOUT JUDGMENT

"What makes it tough for moms during this period," says Best, "is that there's this initial gut reaction to the experience, and then mothers can judge themselves for having those feelings." I know it's not easy, but let yourself feel whatever you are feeling. Those are your feelings, and they don't mean anything about the kind of mom you will be or how much you love your baby. They are just an understandable response to a hard time.

KNOW THAT IT IS NOT YOUR FAULT

When you are doing everything "right" and yet you are still suffering, you might think, *What am I doing wrong?* The answer is *nothing.* "There is this myth that you can control your pregnancy," says Best. But it bears repeating: growing a human being is an incredibly complicated, difficult task. Things go wrong, and much of it is beyond our control. "Talk to your OB or midwife about the actual causes of your complication. In these situations, straight facts can help soothe," says Best.

ADDRESS WHATEVER EMOTIONS YOU ARE HAVING SPECIFICALLY

"Get in touch with whatever you are feeling—guilt, embarrassment, sadness, anger, anxiety, or a cocktail of all of those emotions," recommends Best. "Then care for those feelings in a really specific way. If you feel angry, you could write an angry letter to the circumstances of your pregnancy, to your gestational diabetes. If you feel that you've lost out on something you wanted or deserved, consider giving yourself permission to grieve it. Think through or share with a friend the experiences you wish that you had, acknowledging that fantasy has passed, almost like a eulogy."

FEELING ANXIOUS TOTALLY MAKES SENSE

Best tends to see more anxiety (rather than depressive symptoms) in women who are experiencing pregnancy complications, and that makes sense. One way it might come up, says Best, is what mental health experts call *catastrophizing*, or going to the worst-case scenario in your head.

If you find yourself constantly doing so, Best suggests thinking about other ways things could unfold. "You're helping your brain to remember that 'yeah, the worst-case scenario could happen, but the best-case scenario could also happen . . . and the medium-case scenario.' Remind your mind that there are other options."

UNFORTUNATELY, OTHER PEOPLE MAY NOT GET IT

"There is all this messaging about what pregnancy is supposed to be," says Best. "And in our culture in general, there is a whitewashing of distress, so we don't have good ways of being with someone who is in distress. We just want to help them feel better." So your friends and family may try to cheer you up or even minimize what you are going through in an effort to avoid sitting with you in your distress. That can feel very isolating, but there are things you can do to find support.

How to Feel Supported When You Are Having a Difficult Pregnancy
- **Find one nonjudgmental friend or family member** whom you trust and enlist them to help you. Ask that friend not to dismiss your concerns or minimize them, but listen. If you like to take action in times of

anxiety, ask that friend to help you brainstorm and execute some small ways you can get support and feel more in control of your circumstances, like setting up a Meal Train (Mealtrain.com) and sending the link out for you.

- **Find a care provider you trust and listen to them.** "Give them the job of the hard medical calls," says Best. "Maternal fetal medicine experts have a lot of training, and—let's be real—malpractice is expensive," says Best. "They don't want things to go the wrong way either; their livelihood and reputation rest on it going the right way."
- **Do not Google.** I repeat. Do not Google. Repeat after me: "I will not Google." "Googling never actually helps anyone," says Best.
- **Come up with contingency plans** in the event you need to deliver early or have to be admitted to the hospital. Have neighbors lined up for childcare and friends on deck to cook meals (see "Set Yourself Up for Support" on page 106 for more ideas on how to prepare). Putting some plans in place will help you regain a little sense of control and an idea of how you will cope.
- **Try a little healthy distraction** like going to a movie with a friend or bingeing on a Netflix series.
- **Connect with people who understand what you are going through** (see page 376) online or in person.
- **Know that you are in good company.** Yes, there are the pregnant ladies who look like they are sailing through this thing, but they may be struggling in ways you cannot see, and there are lots of tough mamas

out there gutting it out through a pregnancy that is much harder than they expected. And they, like you, are doing it.

Been There, Done That: Moms Talk About the Emotions of Pregnancy Complications and Being "High Risk"

I have epilepsy, so my pregnancy planning was quite deliberate. I selected a specific seizure medication that has the fewest documented instances of [birth defects]. I chose to stop another medication I had been taking. I began taking prescription folic acid supplements six months in advance. I changed insurers in order to work with specific providers.

—Rebekah, Parker, Colorado

I was a gestational diabetic. I controlled it with diet and exercise, but overall it felt like an incredible failure. Like my body was conspiring to hurt my baby. The education at the hospital I gave birth at was incredibly poor, and I was made to feel as if it was my fault that I'd developed the disorder. I was also really angry that the last few months of my "joyous" pregnancy experience was taken from me by needle sticks, food logs, beeping glucose meters, and weekly check-ins with my neonatal specialist. I felt deprived and like I was being punished, but also terribly anxious that my body was hurting my baby. It turned out fine in the end, but it caused me a whole lot of undue stress.

—Kendra, Atlanta, Georgia

Because I was on complete bed rest for five months, it was hard to depend on other people for food, housework, rides, and so on. I hired help where I could but had to learn to ask friends and family for help. I meditated when I could bear it. I watched a lot of TV—funny stuff.

—ELIZABETH, ATLANTA, GEORGIA

I had terrible hyperemesis gravidarum [severe nausea and vomiting]. Every pregnancy is different, but usually somewhere there is a bump in the road. Don't be sucked in by the "glowing pregnancy" myth and feel less as a result.

—SORREL, LONDON, UK

Planning for Co-Parenting

My husband and I talked about a lot of things before becoming parents—our values, what kinds of parents our parents had been, and how that informed the kinds of parents we wanted to be. Those were good and important conversations and helped us get on the same page about some overarching themes of parenting.

But you know what we did not discuss? Which parent would be in charge of pediatrician visits. Who would handle researching the best way to introduce solid foods. And, down the road, which parent would take the lead on communicating with teachers. And oh so much more! If there is one thing I would love to go back and redo, it is being very specific about how parenting duties were going to be shared. Let my mistake be a boon to you. Here's what I wish I knew.

THINK ABOUT WHAT YOU EACH NEED TO FEEL COMFORTABLE HEADING INTO PARENTING

My brother was born when I was ten years old, so, I had a pretty high level of comfort with babies. My husband, not so much. When we looked over the possible classes we could take before delivery—breastfeeding, childbirth, and so on—he was very interested in a class called Newborn 101. I thought it was a waste of time, but I agreed to go because it seemed to matter so much to him.

All I remember learning from the class is that newborns look weird when they come out (gray and slimy as opposed to pink and shiny), and you don't need to bathe them very often. Afterward, I told my husband it had been a waste of time, because we didn't learn much. "I know!" he said happily. "I feel so relieved." For him, learning that being around a baby is way less complicated than he thought it was going to be was a major stress reliever. I didn't realize until that moment that he had concerns about parenthood that were totally different from mine.

WORK AS A TEAM FROM THE START

When there's a pregnancy involved, the birth parent is intimately involved with parenthood from the start by carrying the baby, but if the non-birth parent can take on some responsibilities during pregnancy, it sets the stage for co-parenting equity down the road.

When Sheehan David Fisher, PhD, assistant professor of psychiatry and behavioral sciences at the Feinberg School of Medicine in Chicago, works with new parents and parents-to-be, he recommends that the non-birth parent stays engaged throughout pregnancy by attending all the prenatal visits, reading books about child development, understanding the changes a developing fetus is going through, spending time around (and holding!) babies, and looking for dads' or parents' meetings to start attending in pregnancy (see page 365). "The more engagement during pregnancy, the better the involvement outcomes in the postpartum," says Fisher.

LOOK AT THE BIG PICTURE OF CO-PARENTING

"I think people can be great dads, but that doesn't necessarily mean they are great co-parents," says Jill Krause, creator of the popular blog *Baby Rabies*. Krause tells parents to "talk with your partner about what it is to be a co-parent versus what it is to be a mom or dad." And set up the expectation early that you will share not only the practical responsibilities of raising a tiny human (like who handles the inputs—food—and who handles the outputs—diapers) but the big decisions that come with being a parent.

"We talked about a birth plan, how we were going to diaper them, and where they were going to sleep." But Krause recommends thinking even bigger than that and talking about other issues you will eventually face in parenting, like managing social media, asking about firearms in the home before sending a child on a playdate, getting help if your kid needs it with school. Not that you have to answer those questions now, but by talking now, you are setting up your "team game plan" for sharing the small and the large aspects of parenting. "Talk about all the issues together so that it doesn't feel like one person is the boss and the other is the employee."

BREAK IT DOWN—IN DETAIL

Fisher meets with parents before delivery to sort out who is going to do what in the days and weeks after birth. Making those kinds of decisions in the moment—when you're feeling overwhelmed and sleep deprived—is much harder. Fisher has folks come up with a plan of who will handle some of the early tasks, including making sure there are groceries and diapers in the home, bathing the baby, and putting him or her down to sleep. If one parent is breastfeeding, then the other can commit to picking the baby up when she starts to cry and bringing her to the breastfeeding parent along with a glass of water and a snack, for instance.

When sleep specialist Kathryn Lee, RN, was researching how to help new parents get better sleep, she actually had them sign a contract listing out which responsibilities they would each take on.

Whether or not you go the contract-writing route, putting to paper a brainstorm of all you will need to do and assigning responsibilities will make it so much easier to share the work when the time comes and also be a great reference when the inevitable arguments about who's working harder begin. And, of course, it will be a living document that changes as you learn more about what parenting actually entails.

I really wish my husband and I had done that so that he could have had ownership over certain aspects of parenting from the get-go. We have a general belief in equity, but I retained so much control over the logistics of parenting that I was usually asking for "help" and then having to turn over reams of information in order for him to follow through. But writing this section of my book has helped me begin to change that dynamic—ten years later. It's never too late, but starting early is *way* better!

In a piece in *The Huffington Post* a few years ago, the blogger M. Blazoned coined a term for the kind of parenting setup my husband and I inadvertently started off with: "The Default Parent:"

> *Default parents know the names of their kids' teachers, all of them. They fill out endless forms, including the 20-page legal document necessary to play a sport at school, requiring a blood oath not to sue when your kids [get] concussions, because they are going to get concussions. They listen to long, boring, intricate stories about gym games that make no sense. They spell words, constantly. They know how much wrapping paper there is in the house. The default parent doesn't have her own calendar, but one with everyone's events on it that makes her head hurt when she looks at it. They know a notary. They buy poster board in 10-packs. They've worked tirelessly to form a bond with the school receptionists. They know their kids' sizes, including shoes, dammit.*

It's exhausting just to read that paragraph, let alone live it. Which is why I suggest taking some time now to consciously set up a fair division of labor. Of course, it will change over time, as you each develop different interests and competencies in parenting and as the hours of your paying jobs ebb and flow. But by starting parenthood with a plan to truly share the tasks in those early weeks and months, you will be laying the groundwork for meaningful co-parenting down the road.

LET THE OTHER PARENT MAKE DECISIONS
AND MISTAKES

Fisher encourages couples to work against the "default parent" setup by making sure both parents have a chance to carve their own path for taking care of the baby without micromanaging each other.

"If somebody feels incompetent or is criticized, they stop trying," says Fisher. "If every time the baby is crying, a dad hands off the baby, it sets up the expectation that mom is the one always solving problems," says Fisher. "I encourage couples to avoid that."

Krause puts a finer point on it: "It does nobody any good for a mom to take on a martyr role or play into stereotypes. You have to give the non-birth parent more credit, show that you trust them and believe they can do this. Allow them to make mistakes, because you're going to make them too, and the last thing you need to do is be at each other's throats when you do."

Been There, Done That: Moms Talk About What They Did to Prepare for Co-Parenting

---

We talked a lot about wanting it to be equal. I was up front about wanting to have the baby because I was pretty sure it was the only way our kid would like me—kids just always love my wife. We took turns getting up at night and still do. We take turns letting the other person sleep in on weekend mornings. We split the evening time so that one of us does pajamas and teeth brushing while the other does

*books and bed, and whoever puts her to bed gets her up in
the morning.* —AMANDA, DECATUR, GEORGIA

*In the first few weeks, my husband was great about letting
me sleep (bottle-feeding helped with that). We shared many
of the responsibilities that come with a newborn. Once he
went back to work and I was still on leave, things shifted
more to me, which made sense, but the tension grew. My
suggestion for new parents is figure out your agreement ahead
of time. Are you going to take turns throughout the night? Do
you get up Monday, Wednesday, and Friday and he takes
Tuesday and Thursday? Does he get up with you? I feel like if
we had done that, we would have saved a lot of energy.*

—AMBER, INDIANAPOLIS, INDIANA

*Next time, I would devise a plan with my husband and
delegate who was doing what. I would insist that he be in
charge of some of the research and decisions. You look into
how we should start solid foods. You decide how we introduce the dogs to the baby. You make a meal plan and cook for
the week.* —JAMIE, ATLANTA, GEORGIA

*Pregnancy is only nine months; parenthood lasts forever!
Use this time to talk to your partner about ideals, wishes,
hopes, values, discipline, expectations, memories of your own
childhood, and how to craft a life together as a new family.*

—REBECCA

Building Your Village

I n almost every interview I conducted for this book, when I asked experts what moms need to do to take care of their mental health, the one word that came up time and again was *support*. That old African proverb "It takes a village to raise a child" is right. This is not a solitary endeavor, nor was it ever meant to be. If you need proof, let me kick a little evolutionary science your way.

Here's how the math of raising a human breaks down among people still living as hunter-gatherers much as our ancestors must have when humans were evolving, according to anthropologist Sarah Hrdy, PhD, author of *Mothers and Others: The Evolutionary Origins of Mutual Understanding*. A child needs to consume thirteen million calories between the day he is born and when he becomes an adult and is able to provide for himself. Since the time between births tends to be shorter in humans than in other apes (close to three to four years), mothers will give birth to a new infant long before her older offspring are anywhere near independence. In fact, the peak nutritional demands for brain development occur around four to five years old, just as mothers would be nursing a new—and very dependent—baby. That means well before a child is able to feed him- or herself, his mother will be busy breastfeeding another infant and will not be able to provide all the calories her older child needs to survive.

So how, then, were we able to get the nutrients we needed to become big-brained humans capable of following that complicated paragraph of evolutionary math? Group members other than parents ("alloparents") filled in. They were sisters, aunts, cousins, and even some non-kin. They were—and remain today—any member of a group who is not a genetic parent that helps care for a child. "Human beings could not have evolved unless mothers had had allomaternal support," says Hrdy. In other words, it takes a village. Let's start building yours.

WHO WILL BE HELPFUL AFTER DELIVERY? AND WHO WON'T BE?

The question is not "Who wants to visit after you give birth?" or "Who lives closest to you?" The question is "Who will be the most helpful?" Think about who has been a support to you in the past. What family members or friends, on the other hand, are more likely to show up when you're having a hard day and ask what's for supper? This is one time (the first of many, I hope) in your life that what matters most is what *you* need and which people will help you meet those needs.

I suggest getting concretely organized about this. Make a list of family and friends (you never have to show it to them, and I promise not to tell them you did it) and write down which ones are likely to show up and cook you a meal, which ones are more likely to want to be entertained while you hold the baby, which ones you are comfortable being in front of in your bathrobe with spit-up on your shoulder. Who will change a diaper? Who can see your messy house? Who wouldn't mind being asked to do some dishes? Who gives really good back rubs? Which friend is likely to share how she raised a child that eats nothing but kale and quinoa? This is not a list of who is better than whom. It's a list of people's strengths and, yes, weaknesses, that will help you figure out who is best to help you when.

A friend who hates to do dishes but is super fun to vent with over a glass of wine is likely someone you'll want to see maybe a month after birth and not in those first few weeks of survival. A mom friend who seems to have it all together might be a terrible choice when you are a weepy new mom but would be terrific support when you have your sea legs and are ready for some tips. In those early weeks, you need friends and family who have supported you through hard times, who don't have high standards for appearance or etiquette, and who will roll up their sleeves and pitch in.

MAKE A SCHEDULE

Once you've got a sense of which friends and family might support you best during different phases of your recovery, map out an ideal scenario of who would visit you when. If your mom is your best friend and your sister can be a stress, then your mom gets to take the first visitor shift. And you can extend an offer to your sister that will make sure she comes later but still feels included. Don't double book folks, and do everything you can to put people up in other people's homes, at motels or hotels, apartment rentals—anywhere other than your house. Unless, of course, your best friend has offered to do some night shifts with the baby or your mom will hold the baby all day while you sleep and shower—then open up the sofa bed and welcome them over.

PRACTICE ASKING FOR WHAT YOU WANT NOW

It's not easy telling your mother-in-law you don't want her in the delivery room or asking that your mom stay at a hotel. Few of us are comfortable with those kinds of conversations, but to embark on parenthood is to embark on a journey of setting boundaries with yourself, with your children, with others. And one of the unexpected and great things about parenthood is that it can give you permission to stand up for what you need. It may not feel comfortable, but practicing in small ways now can make it much easier to continue setting boundaries when the hormones have kicked in, you're sleep deprived, and your little bundle of joy likes to wail her head off from 5:00 to 7:00 each night.

MAKE IT EASY FOR OTHERS TO PITCH IN

People get excited about babies. Remember how they couldn't stop touching your belly or asking your due date? They just want to be a part of it! And guess what? After delivery is a time when they truly can be. Yay! So remember that when people say, "What can I do?" "Let me know if you need anything," and "Call anytime," they mean it. And you should take them up on it by having very concrete ways they can follow through. Even better if you can designate a friend to help you set this up and spread the word for you!

Easy Ways to Help People Help You

- **Create an online shopping list** of nutrient-dense staples you will want to have in your house after the baby arrives.
- **Set up a Care or Google calendar** where people can sign up to help with childcare or pitch in around the house. This is especially important if your partner is not at home with you or you are a solo mom.
- **Set up a meal schedule** through websites such as Mealtrain.com and Takethemameal.com so your friends and family can sign up to bring you dinner.
- **Write up a list of your favorite takeout places** so you can share them with people who want to come visit the baby (they can bring dinner and meet a cute baby—win-win!).
- **Research cleaning services** and ask for gift certificates to use them.
- **Buy a passel of paper plates and plastic cutlery** so friends (and you sometimes) can help set up and break down meals quickly.
- **Hire a bouncer.** Pick someone to help you set boundaries with others when you can't or don't want to. This could be a partner or a close friend; the only qualification for the job is comfort with saying a variation of this as often as needed: "I'm so sorry, Aunt Edna, but right now is just a big time of adjustment for the new family. I know you're so excited for your bridge club to meet little Jimmy, but let's look at next month for a visit."

Set Yourself Up for Support

- **Find new moms'/parents' groups in your area** (see page 374 for information on all kinds of moms' groups).
- **Hire a postpartum doula or night nurse** if finances allow. Or ask for donations as a baby shower gift or put a donation jar by the door and offer it as a concrete way people can help when they visit.
- **Join your local YMCA** so you can start to use the childcare as soon as your child is old enough. You don't even have to work out; you can just find a chair to sit in and read or sleep or shower.
- **Hire a "mommy's helper,"** usually a neighborhood kid who is not old enough to babysit but young enough to be willing to do some household jobs for a very reasonable fee.
- **Make freezer meals** in your third trimester, so you have something quick to heat up and eat in the early weeks.

Twelve Answers to the Question "How Can I Help?"

- Bring a meal when you come over.
- Do a quick cleanup of the kitchen.
- Change the kitty litter.
- Hold this bundle of joy while I take a nap.
- Walk the dog.
- Give the bathroom a once-over.

- Change the sheets.
- Take out the diaper pail.
- Run to the store and pick up *X*, *Y*, and *Z*.
- Sit down and listen to what I am feeling right now.
- Let me just vent for ten minutes!
- Donate to the night nurse / babysitting / cleaning service fund.

DON'T THINK OF IT AS ASKING FOR HELP

Asking for help gets a bad rap. Some of us think it makes us weak. Others worry they are imposing and don't want to be a bother. Still others don't like other folks up in their business. I get all of that. So let's not call this *asking for help*. Let's assume that the evolutionary biologists know what they are talking about when they affirm that alloparents were essential for the survival and development of the human species. Think of all the things suggested in this chapter as nurturing your community, deepening your connections, fostering your friendships, and building your village, one that will not only strengthen you and your family but your whole community, and, dare I say it, the world!

Been There, Done That: Moms Share Stories of Setting Themselves Up for Support After the Baby Arrived

---

We organized a schedule of family coming to help in the first weeks; that was great for getting me out of the house and helping me not feel isolated, since my husband returned to

work quickly after the birth. I also stocked the freezer with casseroles at the end of the third trimester.

—COLLEEN, BROOKLYN, NEW YORK

Get a night nurse! Best money spent ever. I saved for months for it, and as a single mom, it was critical.

—KYM

Limit visitors to thirty minutes.

—JACKIE, DECATUR, GEORGIA

I recommend that solo moms do whatever they can to secure paid help—reliable paid help. Reallocate funds, save during pregnancy, ask for money instead of gifts for the baby shower.   —DOMENICA, BROOKLYN, NEW YORK

My advice would be not to host anyone unless they offer to help a lot, and never feel obligated to do hostess-like things. Have people visit you for twenty minutes at a time and feel free to make them visit you while you're in your own bed if you've had a C-section. You shouldn't have to get up.

—STEPHANIE, ILLINOIS

I am glad my mother came out to visit right after the birth because I did need the help. However, it was a challenging time. A lot of mothers seem to find it stressful when their daughters have a child. My mother was stressing out over things like the cleanliness of my house, when I was just in survival mode. I have friends who also felt like their mothers became unusually intense or judgmental at this time.   —RACHEL, PENNSYLVANIA

I wish I'd set clearer boundaries that what I really wanted was help with tasks like cooking, dishes, and occasional baby care, but that I only wanted advice if I asked for it directly. The unsolicited advice was a real source of friction and undermined my confidence.

—CARRIE, SAINT PAUL, MINNESOTA

Preparing to Feed Your Child in a Way That Works for You

This book will not be extolling the virtues of one type of feeding over another. That's been covered one million times already. What I do want to do is support you in making a choice that feels good for you, offer tips on how to set yourself up for a smooth start in whatever method you choose and prepare for—and move through—the difficulties that can arise. I want to make sure you have the support and information you need to feed your child with comfort and confidence.

WHY THE HIGH STAKES OF BREASTFEEDING?

There is no doubt that breastfeeding is a great choice for feeding your baby, and that is a good message to have out there. But what *is* wrong is equating whether or not a mom breastfeeds with who she is as a mom, and that's exactly what society does *all the time*. We have to get deep for a moment to see how we ended up at that false conclusion.

"Most of our lives are devoted to preventing risks of all kinds," says Joan Wolf, PhD, author of *Is Breast Best? Taking*

On the Breastfeeding Experts and the New High Stakes of Parenthood. "We have this ethos that if we just think hard enough and get the right information we should be able to prevent risk. This is extremely problematic as a way of being, because it's not possible. And it's certainly problematic as a way to approach motherhood, because it is crazy making."

That's an important overall point about motherhood that I will explore more in the final section of this book, but here let's just address the intersection between risk culture and breastfeeding. "In our culture, being healthy is seen as a manifestation of your choices," says Wolf. "If you are not healthy, it has to do with what you didn't do. If you are healthy, it is because you made good decisions." In reality, our health is a result of a complex set of factors, including genetics and environment, and what you eat is only one small part of it. But, Wolf argues, it is often portrayed as the definitive determinant of health.

"The breastfeeding controversy fits very well into that," says Wolf, "because we like to think that what we eat determines what our health is." And there's another layer that gets added in, what Wolf calls "the ideology of total motherhood, which essentially tells women they are 100 percent responsible for the products they produce." Put those two together and—whammo!—there is one heck of lot of pressure to breastfeed that leaves women who choose not to or women who are unable to feeling like they have failed at one of the first tests of motherhood. But they have not. Society has failed mothers by not offering them support in feeding their babies in the best way for them and their families.

EXPLORE WHAT FEELS RIGHT TO YOU

"This is one of the issues where you need to really dig deep and decide what's most important for you," says Karen Kleiman, LCSW, founder of the Postpartum Stress Center in Rosemont, Pennsylvania. "Don't let messages from the media or relatives tell you what to do."

That's easier said than done, of course, for all the reasons outlined above. "It is difficult in this environment to make a truly unencumbered choice," says Suzanne Barston, author of *Bottled Up: How the Way We Feed Babies Has Come to Define Motherhood and Why It Shouldn't.* "I think the best thing to do is to take all the medical and scientific reasons out of it for one minute. Most pediatricians agree that both breastfeeding and formula-feeding will adequately feed your child. Then talk factually and emotionally about what breastfeeding will mean for you."

Barston recommends sitting down and writing a brain dump about feeding your child. What are all the things that come to mind when you think about breastfeeding? How about formula-feeding? "Look at the list and see what preconceived notions you have, where your values and desires fall, and what concerns you have that can be addressed.

BREAK AWAY FROM *EITHER-OR*

One of the downsides of the high-stakes world of baby feeding is that it is often presented as an all-or-nothing proposition. "So many of us go in thinking it's exclusive breastfeeding or bust," says Barston. "Instead, if you can go in with less rigid belief systems in place, it allows you to be a little more flexible and very often allows you to come up with some kind of combination of the two that works great."

BE OPEN TO THINGS CHANGING

So much (all of?) parenting cannot be predicted until you have lived through it, and breastfeeding is a great example of that. You may feel very strongly that you want to breastfeed exclusively for the first year of your child's life and then discover you can't stand pumping at work and opt for some kind of breast/formula combination. You may believe breastfeeding is the *only* way to feed a child and then discover that you really don't like doing it or encounter problems that make it impossible. Or the opposite can happen.

"When I went to the OB forty years ago, he asked if I wanted to breastfeed. I told him, 'I don't see myself as a breast-feeding kind of person,'" remembers Kleiman. "He told me to do it for a few days and 'if you don't like it, stop.' That sounded reasonable, so I put my baby to my breast and decided I never wanted to do anything else."

Allowing yourself the room to change your mind and being open to the possibility that circumstances could change the way you feed your baby from the way you planned to will help you adjust if you need to.

That said, a little preparation will go a long way in helping you achieve *your* goals with greater ease and comfort.

HOW TO PREPARE FOR BREASTFEEDING

Despite all the emphasis on breastfeeding, one important fact that is usually left out is that breastfeeding is a learned skill, and few of us receive any education on it before trying to do it ourselves. Back in the days of our ancestors, we would have watched our mothers and sisters and aunts and friends breastfeed before we tried it ourselves, and we would have had them all around us as we embarked on the endeavor. Nowadays, with smaller families spread farther apart, most of us are flying solo with little to no support in those first few awkward days or weeks of learning how to feed a tiny person with our bodies. And, by the way, your baby is learning too. So here are some things you can do to help both of you.

TAKE A PRENATAL BREASTFEEDING CLASS

"This is one of the most important things you can do," says Ayelet Kaznelson, an internationally board-certified lactation consultant in Manhattan. "Research shows that women who take a prenatal class have better breastfeeding outcomes." In a class, you can learn practical, direct advice on the basics of breastfeeding, like how to establish a good latch. But you can also share any concerns or fears you have, learn a little bit about what to expect as you begin breastfeeding, and what signs you should watch for that mean you should get professional support sooner rather than later. "Almost every situation and complication can be dealt with," says Kaznelson. "Most of the time, with a good amount of support and help, you can get through them."

- **Watch the video** *Follow Me Mum,* a terrific (albeit very dated) video on breastfeeding that can help you start off with a good latch from feed one.
- **Choose a "baby-friendly" hospital.** This is a designation bestowed by UNICEF and the WHO that is given to hospitals that do certain things to promote breastfeeding, such as allowing babies to room in with moms and not handing out formula packs without a request.
- **Consider having a doula for labor** who also supports women postpartum and is a certified lactation consultant.
- **Attend any breastfeeding classes** offered by the hospital or birthing center after you deliver and have the lactation consultant on call visit you so you can ask all your questions and get started with a good latch.
- **Find a lactation consultant you like** so you can reach out if you have difficulty once you return home (or in the hospital if you need to). Look for a consultant who is internationally board certified. That means she will have *IBCLC* after her name and will have completed a year of coursework, 1,500 clinical hours, and a daylong exam. "Phone them up and ask them what their opinions are on feeding and infant care and find who clicks with you, then you'll know who to call if you need to," says Carrie Bruno, IBCLC, who runs the Mama Coach in Calgary, Canada.
- **Research breastfeeding clinics or groups in your area.** Kaznelson recommends seeing if there is an

ongoing breastfeeding class in your area that operates more like a new moms' group. You can meet weekly with a certified lactation consultant, troubleshoot, and (bonus!) make new mom friends. Plus, no one will care if your baby (or you) is crying and your boobs are hanging out.

- **Know that you will have a learning curve** with breastfeeding and that there will be ups and downs. "Nursing can feel like a bit of a roller-coaster ride," says Bruno. "There's ups and downs. One feed you think, *I got this, we're good.* And the next feed you may think, *I can't do this, it isn't working, he's not getting anything.* But you should see an upward trend. Within two weeks, quite often you will feel good about it, your baby will be getting food, and you're not having tenderness.'"

- **See if your insurance will cover lactation support and/or a breast pump.** Some internationally board-certified lactation consultants accept insurance for visits at home or at your pediatrician's office. Call your health insurance to see what they offer and if they have a list of consultants with whom they work. Research and buy a breast pump.

Breastfeeding When You Are a Survivor of Assault

One circumstance that can make breastfeeding especially difficult is if you are a survivor of physical (particularly sexual) assault. That doesn't mean you cannot breastfeed if you want to, says Kathleen Kendall-Tackett, PhD, an internationally board-certified lactation consultant in Amarillo, Texas. Plenty of moms who are survivors of assault go on to love breastfeeding. In a study Kendall-Tackett conducted of 6,410 new mothers, survivors of sexual assault breastfed at exactly the same rate as other moms. But breastfeeding can bring up emotions, feelings, or memories that are painful and for which you deserve support. There are great resources for finding professional support and for connecting with other women who have had similar experiences (see page 365). Kendall-Tackett offers this general advice:

Give yourself space. For some mothers, jumping right into skin-to-skin contact may feel too intense, and that's okay. Start with a blanket or other material over your body and ease into it a bit at a time.

Talk with your birth and pediatric providers. If you're comfortable, share your history and your concerns to ensure you will have compassionate support from them.

Recognize that you may not love breastfeeding. And that's okay too. Women's responses range from loving to hating it. If you don't like it, be clear in your mind about why you want to continue—or don't. If you're having a fixable problem, seek skilled care from a lactation specialist.

Know that many other women have experienced the challenges you face. You are not alone in this. Reach out in your communities or online. You'll find many have walked this same road and can offer you the best support and advice (see page 365).

HOW TO PREPARE FOR FORMULA-FEEDING

Suzanne Barston literally wrote the book (and the blog) on formula-feeding. She intended to breastfeed her first baby and ended up switching to formula after a serious struggle with breastfeeding and postpartum depression related to breastfeeding difficulties (and all the pressure she and others had put on her). She went on to launch a blog, *Fearless Formula Feeder*, to support formula-feeding moms and eventually became a certified lactation counselor so she could launch a feeding consultant business that would enable her to support moms through whatever way they planned to feed their babies. Here are her tips for preparing for formula-feeding.

- **Own your choice.** "If you've done your prenatal 'homework' and read up on both breastfeeding and bottle-feeding, you can feel confident that you're making the best choice for you and your family, not the family in the room next to yours."
- **Have an advocate.** When you're exhausted from giving birth, possibly in pain, and those postpartum hormones are pulsing through you, it may not be easy to stand up for yourself if someone questions your choice. So designate a person—your partner, doula, or a friend—to calmly share that you plan to formula-feed if the topic comes up. She also suggests creating a written document to post above your bed that says, "I've made an informed decision to bottle-feed and ask that my choice be respected. Thank you for your cooperation." This is especially

important if you are delivering in a hospital that has been designated "baby-friendly" for its practices to promote breastfeeding.

• **Come prepared.** Some hospitals will only provide formula when it is requested and in one "dose" at a time. Bring your own supply to have on hand so you can respond to your baby's hunger cues without having to wait on someone else. Plus, you will get to bring the brand you have researched and chosen rather than being stuck with the hospital brand. Barston recommends single-use, ready-to-feed packs, which are available from most commercial formula companies.

• **Look into the low-cost options.** Many formula companies provide coupons and sample packs, so Barston recommends signing up for coupons on brand websites and having your relatives and friends do the same. WIC (the Women, Infants, and Children nutrition program run by the USDA) offers subsidized formula to women who qualify.

• **Bond through bottle-feeding.** "There is a lot you can do to make bottle-feeding a close bonding experience," advises Barston. If you are comfortable with it, start skin on skin (and that can go for anyone in the family who is feeding the baby, including siblings). "The baby can be in her diaper, and you take your shirt off," says Barston. "Hold them close, make sure you make eye contact and are responsive to your baby's reactions during the feeding."

• **Research new moms' groups that are not organized around breastfeeding.** Many postnatal groups focus on breastfeeding or are made up largely of women who are breastfeeding. That can feel very alienating if you are not. Look for moms' groups that are focused more on general camaraderie and acceptance of all choices. (See page 258.)

- **Choose a supportive pediatrician.** One of your best resources, says Barston, is a supportive pediatrician who can help you figure out the specifics of types of formula, amounts, and approaches and help you troubleshoot when you run into difficulty. When you interview pediatricians, share your plan to bottle-feed and ask if they will be supportive of your choice. If they won't, look for another provider.

- **Check out online bottle-feeding support and information** like *Fearless Formula Feeder* on Facebook or the formula-friendly message boards on JustMommies.com. You can also find several guides to using formula on HealthyChildren.org, run by the American Academy of Pediatrics.

- **Prepare for people asking why you are not breastfeeding** and even trying to convince you why you should or make you feel bad that you aren't. You don't owe anyone an explanation, but staring blankly back at people can make for awkward social moments, so Barston recommends having some responses like, "Formula-feeding is right for us," at the ready. You can even let people know "I've done the research and feel really good about how my family is planning to feed our baby." Or whatever feels right to you.

REMEMBER THIS IS YOUR CHOICE NO MATTER WHAT OTHERS SAY

Whatever feeding choice you make, you may feel pressure from others to choose a different approach. "I have moms who feel like they're letting their own hippie mom down by bottle-feeding and moms whose relatives think it's ridiculous that she's pumping when she could be sleeping," says New York City psychotherapist Sarah Best. "Knowing your own values and making the choice that best serves you is the best armor against any judgment that will inevitably come."

Been There, Done That: Moms Share How They Planned to Feed

I wanted to breastfeed, and I had to hire a lactation consultant to make it work. She was wonderful and worth every cent. —STEPHANIE, ILLINOIS

I planned to formula-feed. I knew I would only be taking six weeks off and didn't want the extra stress of trying to nurse (on top of being a new mom). I was unsure how I would adjust to motherhood and decided to take this one off my plate. I researched types of formula as well as prep and storage information. I also read about what to do if confronted by a pushy or judgmental person in the hospital or at the doctor's office. Being prepared help me feel that I could give my answers more confidently. —LAURA, PENNSYLVANIA

We prepared by taking a class on breastfeeding, and I spent lots of time talking to a close friend who was breastfeeding while I was pregnant.

—Elizabeth, Saint Paul, Minnesota

I knew I wanted to exclusively formula-feed since before I got pregnant. I read anything I could find online about different formulas, bottles, is it necessary to sterilize, do I need a warmer, and so on. Fearless Formula Feeder *was very helpful to me, as was the book* Bottled Up. *I made sure we were stocked and ready to go before baby got here.*

—Amber, Indianapolis, Indiana

I knew I wanted to breastfeed or at least try. I honestly thought I would hate it because I hated having my nipples touched. Turns out I loved breastfeeding.

—Dominga, Saint Paul, Minnesota

I planned to formula-feed. I spoke extensively with my doctor (and my friends in an attempt to head off judgment) about it. I researched formula and bottles and had everything sterilized and waiting for our return home from the hospital.   —Amanda, San Diego, California

Bottle-feeding was an amazing experience for me from the very first bottle I gave my daughter. We would make ourselves comfortable on the sofa or in bed and take our time, maybe listening to soothing music whilst feeding. I always enjoyed feeding her and never felt like she, or I, were missing out on anything. If there is any other mum out there who is thinking about choosing to bottle-feed her baby, I would simply reassure her and tell her she knows what is best for her baby and that bottle-feeding makes her exactly as good a mum as breastfeeding would.

—Anonymous

Getting Ready for Birth

A birth plan. It sounds like a good idea, right? But when you step back for a moment and consider the biologically monumental task you are undertaking—growing a person inside of you and then pushing him or her out of a rather small opening in your body and into the world—the idea that you can really *plan* for how that will go seems a little bit of a, well, stretch.

Instead, I suggest recasting the idea of a birth plan. Maybe call it a list of birth wishes or birth hopes. Or you could call it your birthing approach. Whatever name you give it (or maybe don't even name it), it's a good idea to build in some flexibility into the way you envision bringing your child into the world. That flexibility will help you adjust if you need to and recover if things do not go as you imagined.

THERE IS NO "BEST" BIRTH

During my first pregnancy, I wanted to have an unmedicated birth. Not because I was worried about an epidural harming my child or me but really just to show that I could. And yet that doesn't make sense given my typical relationship to medication. I take ibuprofen at the whisper of a headache. I grab a Sudafed if I think a cold is coming on. Why was birth different? Because I had internalized the message that giving birth without pharmaceutical pain relief was "better" than giving birth with it.

I was buying into a myth. There is no ideal birth. Or perfect birth. Or best birth. Babies come into this world in all different settings and with all different levels of support all over the world.

And the way your baby enters this world is not a measure of the kind of mother you will be or the priorities you will have or how much you love your child. The way your baby enters this world will be a combination of your particular pregnancy, the things that make you comfortable, the community and setting in which you are giving birth, and the vagaries of nature that make birth the unexpected, miraculous thing that it is. Some of that you have control over and some you don't.

IT IS NOT ALL ON YOU

The problem with a lot of books and articles on this topic is that they sell the idea that if you just make the "right" choices, you can have a certain kind of experience, and that puts the responsibility of the outcome on your shoulders. It is not. Most deliveries in the United States are overseen by a birth professional (ideally, one of your choosing) who is responsible for you and your baby having a healthy birth (the true goal).

"Women are told to just use positive thinking to 'Trust in birth,' and 'Trust your body,'" says Pam England, creator of the Birthing from Within series of childbirth classes whose first birth (intended to be at home) ended in a C-section. This kind of "magical thinking," says England, clashes directly with the medicalized industry of giving birth in the United States in which 40 percent of women are induced and a third of women end up having C-sections. The result? When women have hospital births different from what they had hoped for, they often blame themselves for not trying hard enough, not making the right plans, being "weak," or "failing."

THE MYTH OF NATURAL VERSUS NONNATURAL BIRTH

Giving birth is usually presented as an either-or proposition. Either you will have a "natural" birth or you will have a "medicated" birth, which is implicitly nonnatural. There are at least two problems with this approach. First of all, no matter what happens from the time labor begins until the moment your baby exits your body, you are going to be experiencing a natural process—bringing a living being into the world.

Secondly, this is not a binary proposition. There is a continuum of ways to experience the process, from birthing at home into a tub of warm water to being in an operating room delivering your baby through C-section—and all kinds of possibilities in between. So long as you and your baby are healthy and safe, none of them is "better" than another.

THINK ABOUT HOW *YOU* HAVE FELT
IN OTHER SITUATIONS

One woman's good birth is another's worst-case scenario. Forget about what your best friend or sister did when they gave birth. Toss all the "shoulds" and just start with a little soul-searching about what really matters to you. Here are some questions to start the conversation:

- How do I manage pain?
- How do I feel when I am in a hospital?
- Do I like being surrounded by people?
- Do I like being alone?
- Do I trust medical experts to make the best decision for me?
- Do I feel uncomfortable in medicalized settings?
- Do I use medication to manage pain usually?
- Do I avoid medication as much as possible?
- How do I feel when I am not in control?
- What is most useful to me in times of stress?
- What makes me feel better?
- What makes me feel worse?

KEEP IT SHORT AND FOCUSED

If you are going to write down a birth plan, make it short and focused on the most important thing to you. "Start off by saying, 'My birth plan is to do my very best,'" recommends England. "Then pick one thing that is most important to you and ask for that, like, 'I don't want to be offered drugs every time someone enters the room. I'll ask for drugs if I need them.' The shorter the plan is, the greater the chance your providers will read it and help you work toward it."

PLAN YOUR SUPPORT FOR THE WISHES YOU HAVE

"Pick a provider who supports your desires, but one who not only gives lip service to that but actively encourages you to put in place supports to make that happen," recommends Lauren Abrams, CNM, director of midwifery at Mount Sinai Hospital in Manhattan.

"If you want to have an unmedicated birth, get as much support as you can during labor," says Abrams. If it is financially feasible for you, Abrams says, "the number-one thing you can do to avoid a medicated birth is to get a doula."

The research backs her up according to Emily Oster, PhD, author of *Expecting Better: Why the Conventional Pregnancy Wisdom Is Wrong—and What You Really Need to Know.* In one study, women were randomly assigned a doula when they checked into the hospital, while other women gave birth without one. "Women who were assigned to the doula group had lower levels of epidurals and C-sections," says Oster.

Abrams also recommends that women hoping to avoid medication or other interventions during birth stay away from "tertiary care centers with very high C-section rates" and look for centers that have pain-relieving elements such as warm showers in place. "If you are going to a labor and delivery unit that doesn't even have showers, you are not going to get what you need to have an unmedicated birth," says Abrams.

THINK ABOUT PLANS B AND C

"What you really want is a birth framework," recommends Oster, who, besides researching labor and delivery as an economist, has been through it twice herself. "It's like a game tree: 'If this happens, then this is a choice I want to make,' 'If the following thing arises, then this is what I would like to do.'" Thinking through choices you can make will help you retain a sense of control if things differ from your plans.

Think about the one or two things you hope won't happen, advises England. "Some people are afraid of needles and really don't want an IV; some people are terrified of a long labor."

Then prepare for those possibilities. One of the moms I surveyed ended up with a C-section after hoping for an unmedicated delivery in a birthing center. But she had talked through that possibility with her midwife and doula, and they both stayed with her through the whole process and photographed the birth as they had planned to, which meant a lot to her.

Do you want to learn some breathing techniques to help you adjust if you planned for an epidural but arrived too late to get one? Do you want to come up with a mantra of acceptance when things deviate from your plan? There's no right answer, but exploring how you hope to react in a changing situation will help you be better prepared for it.

If you are able to bring self-compassion (see page 335) "to

that moment," says England, "then you have a different kind of control—control over what you're doing to yourself in your mind, how you're thinking about yourself."

EXPECT UNCERTAINTY

"In our society, everybody has to 'keep their shit together,'" says England. "We want to look good, know what we are doing, be informed, and have everything go exactly as planned. In birth, that isn't what we should be striving for. We should look for the moment when we didn't know what to do, when we didn't know what to expect from ourselves." The very act of being open to uncertainty—expecting it, even—can help it be way less scary if it happens.

WHAT LABOR AND DELIVERY CAN TEACH US ABOUT PARENTING

"This may be our first lesson in how little is under our control when it comes to parenting," says Abrams. "Even with hundreds of years of research in obstetrics, we don't know what starts labor. So it's unpredictable, and you have to sort of get into the mind-set of letting go. It's going to happen when it's going to happen. It's going to be what it's going to be."

"What I would wish for all my clients, friends—everybody I love," says psychotherapist Sarah Best, "is that—as they go into the experience—they stay open to it, flexible, and positive about themselves. Trust the advice of your care providers, and know that you are doing the best you can."

And you can take that quote and apply it to *any* part of the parenting sections ahead.

Preparing for the Legal Logistics of Birth for the LGBTQ Community

Beyond preparing for the way a baby will enter the world, LGBTQ families may have to consider the legal supports they will have in place when it happens—documents that enable the non-birth parent to have hospital visitation rights, make medical decisions, and complete second parent adoptions (if necessary) right away.

"Most of the time, state laws around medical decision-making limit these rights to biological family members," says Morgane Richardson, a birth doula and childbirth educator in New York City. "I tell my clients to make sure their care provider knows who the decision makers are before they give birth." Additionally, Richardson recommends speaking to a lawyer who specializes in LGBTQ family law (see page 366) to make sure you have the documents you need for your family to have full rights in the birthing space. She also tells her clients to read the birth center's or hospital's Patient Bill of Rights and Hospital Bill of Rights, find out if there is an on-staff social worker who can help them prepare for the logistics of delivery, and let the staff know how you would like to be addressed (*Mom*, *Mama*, by your first name?) during delivery and recovery.

Been There, Done That: Moms Share the Plans They Made (or Didn't) for Birth

With the birth of my son, my birth plan didn't get me very far. I was overwhelmed with pain and couldn't find my way to all the things I had learned or prepared for. I had an epidural and then, once I wasn't dizzy with pain, a lovely birth. Second time around, I prepared more, and with a doula who helped me anticipate various possibilities (and pain levels) so that I could have more options available to me during my daughter's birth. With that approach, I was able to deliver without drugs, but both births were amazing experiences with healthy babies at the end.

—DIANA, MONTCLAIR, NEW JERSEY

I laugh about my first birth plan. It was so cute, every single detail planned out. And, as it turned out, the birth went exactly according to my plans. That never happened again. By the time I had my third child, my birth plan was "I'm going to wear mascara."

—ERICA, PITTSBURGH, PENNSYLVANIA

I wrote a note to my midwives explaining that I had difficulty advocating for myself and I would like them to keep asking me if I was comfortable and not to take silence as consent. That was really helpful.

—AMANDA, PORTLAND, OREGON

Get a doula! They are super helpful and supportive. Also, train for your birth. It's like running a marathon. You don't set out to run a marathon without training for it. Treat birth as a huge, intense physical exertion that you need to prepare for with exercise and prenatal yoga.   —ANONYMOUS

I wanted my first delivery to be at a birthing center, and I ended up with a hospital C-section. This was very dis-

appointing and emotionally difficult, but my birth plan did account for what I would want if there was a C-section. It also turned out that having a C-section was a more positive experience than I expected it to be. It meant a lot to me that my midwife and doula still stayed with me and took photos during it. —RACHEL, PENNSYLVANIA

The piece of advice that helped me the most came from one of our birth classes. They said, "Your first goal should be a vaginal birth. If that means you need to take an epidural so you can rest after a long labor, then do it. Your next goal should be to have a healthy baby. So if you need to have a C-section to do it, so be it! The important thing is that at the end of all this, you will go home with your baby, no matter how it comes out." Hearing this from midwives at a birth center was very liberating.

—ALI, PHILADELPHIA, PENNSYLVANIA

Packing Your Emotional
First-Aid Kit

I didn't expect to have postpartum anxiety after the birth of my first daughter, but because I had always had pretty bad mood symptoms when I had PMS, I did do one thing to "prepare" for the possibility. My husband and I agreed that I could say anything I was feeling—even if it was kind of dark and ugly—after giving birth and he would listen to me without judgment and get me help. That's all. That's the one thing we did to prepare for the emotional transition I was about to undergo. But it did serve us well when I experienced debilitating postpartum anxiety after my first daughter was born (see page 208 for more on that story).

After having postpartum anxiety once, I decided to be really prepared for kid number two. Besides keeping in place my husband's and my agreement about being able to say whatever I was feeling, I added several concrete steps that I believe can benefit *everyone*.

- Learn the symptoms of perinatal mood and anxiety disorders that are listed on pages 212–223. Ask your partner or a close friend or family member to read them too.

- Talk to your OB, primary care provider, and pediatrician about how they will help you if you are experiencing mood or anxiety disorder symptoms after delivery and how best to be in touch with them about it.
- Write out a sleep plan that enables you and your partner to get the uninterrupted stretches of sleep that are so critical to emotional health and resilience (see page 174).
- Make a plan to start moving your body in whatever way your physical recovery allows and as soon as it allows.
- Research new moms' groups and meet-ups (see page 374) so you have immediate support and a plan to get out of the house on a regular basis.
- Pick someone—could be your partner, could be your mom or a close friend—with whom you feel completely comfortable and ask them to make the same pact my husband and I did—that you can tell them anything you are feeling, no matter how "crazy" sounding, and, rather than judge you, they will commit to getting you help.
- Bookmark organizations that offer confidential help, including Postpartum Support International (www .postpartum.net), the Postpartum Stress Center (www.postpartumstress.com), and the Seleni Institute (www.seleni.org). See page 367 for more resources.

If You Have a History of a Mood or Anxiety Disorder, Take a Few More Steps:

- Make sure your phone is programmed with professionals such as your OB, primary care doctor, pediatrician, psychotherapist, or psychiatrist, whom you can call from the hospital. After my second daughter's birth, I spoke with both the on-call pediatrician and my psychiatrist and made the choice to take a low-dose antianxiety drug right away.

- If you plan to breastfeed, research the breastfeeding safety of any medications you have used in the past or are currently taking. Two great resources are LactMed and the Infant Risk Center. Both have apps for your phone so you can consult them in your doctors' offices or from the hospital if need be.

These are only a few additions to your packing and preparation list for the hospital, and taking them will do three things for you. One, it will help you internalize one of the main messages of this book—the possibility that you might struggle and that it is okay if you do. Two, it will give you the comfort that if you do feel badly or scared or uncomfortable after your baby is born, you have resources at your fingertips to feel better. Three, it will enable you to begin to feel better and enjoy motherhood so much sooner than if you are completely unprepared for the possibility.

So, while you're packing some comfortable socks, your

robe, and your favorite brand of maxi pads (yes, pack those three things), also create your Emotional First Aid Kit. Because those three benefits are pretty big payoffs for just a little bit of work.

PART II

Starting Strong

Your Guide to Thriving in the First Year

You did it. If you gave birth, you did that thing your body has been preparing for the better part of a year. If you adopted or are fostering, your research, hard work, planning, and preparation helped you bring a new person into your family! You're a mom! Or you've grown your family. What an incredible accomplishment. However things went down, you did it. Your baby is here. Congratulations.

If you are in the hospital with a new baby, you probably want to start reading this section right here. If you are beginning your journey at home, skip to page 153.

If You Are Recovering
in the Hospital

Your body has just been through one of the hardest (*the* hardest?) things it has ever done. You may have been in a very long labor; you may be recovering from surgery. Your body needs rest and sleep right now. Give in to it. Put someone else in charge of the baby (a partner, your mom, the nursery) and let your body fall into a deep sleep. When you wake up from it, if your physical state allows you to, waddle to a warm shower and put on those really comfortable pajamas you packed. Then get back into your bed. Stay put and rest. That is all I ask of you, and that had better be all that anybody else is asking of you.

Here are a few other tips for taking care of yourself in these two to four days of hospital recovery:

GET AHEAD OF PAIN

"Take pain relief if you need it," says Lauren Abrams, CNM, director of midwifery at Mount Sinai Hospital in Manhattan, and take it as directed. Don't wait until the pain is unbearable. It's harder to manage pain once it gets a foothold. Keeping it at bay will help you feel more comfortable.

HAVE PEACEFUL TIME

"After I had my first son, lots of people came to visit me. They were so happy, and I felt so miserable," says Abrams. "I hadn't slept in two days, and people were showing up expecting me to have regular conversations with them. Think of the first twenty-four hours as sacred time for you, your partner, and your baby. Either limit visitors or don't let everyone know right away that the baby has been born," recommends Abrams.

MOVE AROUND WHEN YOU CAN

As soon as you have taken a good long rest and as soon as your recovery and provider allow, try small walks around the recovery ward. "Get out of bed early and move around," says Abrams.

ASK FOR FEEDING SUPPORT

If you are planning to breastfeed, ask that the lactation consultant on call pay you a visit as soon as possible, and attend any classes offered. If the hospital consultant is not available, you can also call someone in (see page 115 for advice on finding a good lactation consultant). If you are formula-feeding, ask the nurses to help you and your partner get those first bottles going.

Been There, Done That: Moms Share Stories and Advice About Those First Few Days in the Hospital

After my first, I didn't want my baby to leave my side. That resulted in no rest and complete anxiety, especially since I had to have a Cesarean, which limits movement after surgery. After I had my second child, I let the nurses take him to the nursery for me to get rest, eat, and shower!

—TIFFANY, HOUSTON, TEXAS

Limit people visiting to either all at once (so it gets done and you can rest) or have just family. Use the staff. Ask tons of questions. If they have a lactation consultant in house, use them! —AMY, HOUSTON, TEXAS

I learned that you can put a note on your door that says, "Sleeping, please come back at 5:00 P.M." (Or you can ask your nurse to do it.) Key.

—MOM TO TWO IN PORTLAND, OREGON

Our family and friends were so excited to meet the baby, and we were happy to share that time with them, but it felt like a revolving door, and I wish we had been more intentional about carving out time for just the three of us.

—AMBER, INDIANAPOLIS, INDIANA

Having visitors is such a subjective decision that every woman needs to be up front with what they want to happen, regardless of what their family and friends want to

happen. Maybe they just want their spouse to be there for the hospital stay, or maybe they want the entire neighborhood. We all need to decide for ourselves.

—CARRIE, ARLINGTON, VIRGINIA

If Your Baby Is in the NICU

Every year, some five hundred thousand babies are treated in the NICU. If your baby is one of them—whether he spends a few days there or has an extended stay—the beginning of your child's life will be a little bit different from what you expected, and you deserve attention and support for that. Research shows that experiencing a NICU stay increases the risk of anxiety, depression, or PTSD (see pages 205–223 for more about these conditions), and even when parents don't develop a mood disorder, they can still experience symptoms of these conditions.

I spoke with Kelli Kelley—the founder and executive director of Hand to Hold (handtohold.org), a nonprofit that supports NICU families—whose two children were born preterm, to find out ways to cope with the stress of a NICU stay.

FIND FAMILIES WHO KNOW WHAT
YOU ARE GOING THROUGH

Hand to Hold does something really amazing. They match you with other NICU parents who have shared the same experience. For instance, if you're a mom of a twenty-nine-weeker, they will connect you with a parent who also had a twenty-nine-weeker and has gone through training in providing peer-to-peer emotional support. "Being able to call or text with a parent who understands what you are going through is critical to processing your emotions," says Kelley.

To get connected with other parents, visit handtohold.org and click "Get Support" or call 855-424-6428. You will be contacted within twenty-four hours. The website also has tons of information to help you manage both the logistical and emotional aspects of this time, along with support for families who experience the loss of their baby. See page 375 for more resources for NICU parents.

OPEN UP ABOUT WHAT YOU ARE FEELING

"It is so important for us to not bottle up our feelings and try to 'move on,'" says Kelley, "that we talk to others and understand and process all the emotions of a NICU stay." The March of Dimes, which has a program to support NICU parents in the hospital, offers this advice (that really should be given to any new mom):

> *Give yourself permission to cry and feel overwhelmed. You may be concerned that if you let your feelings flow, you'll never be able to pull yourself back together. But you will. Allow yourself to feel this release of emotion.*

CONNECT WITH YOUR BABY

Most NICUs now practice kangaroo care, in which parents hold their babies skin to skin, which has been shown to significantly improve the health of premature babies who are learning to regulate their body's systems. It can also really benefit your mental health to feel connected to your baby, says Kelley.

Of course, "it can be overwhelming and scary to hold a baby for the first time when they are hooked up to machines," says Kelley. And there may be situations in which you cannot hold your baby yet. In those instances, Kelley recommends starting with asking to change your baby's diaper. "For a lot of NICU parents, that's the first hug, the first real interaction and touch with the baby." And, says Kelley, "the more we interact with our babies, the more confident caregivers we become."

KNOW THAT A NICU EXPERIENCE
CAN BE TRAUMATIC

The NICU is filled with babies experiencing different levels of health challenges and interventions (especially in hospitals with large NICU units), some life-threatening, others not. Whatever the severity of your family's situation, you will also be experiencing everything that is going on around you for other families. And that involves some trauma, which is why NICU parents are at a higher risk of experiencing post-traumatic stress disorder (PTSD). See page 218 for more on the condition.

MAKE USE OF HOSPITAL SUPPORT

In recent years, there has been an increased awareness of the importance of supporting the mental health of parents in the NICU, and in 2016, the National Perinatal Association released guidelines outlining the mental health support staff and family support programs NICU hospitals should have available.

At the very least, there should be a hospital social worker there to help you manage not only the emotions of this time but also the financial and logistical challenges you are facing. Others have staff psychiatrists or psychologists on hand or have partnered with organizations such as Hand to Hold to provide a more formal support system for NICU parents.

It is especially critical that you reach out for mental health support (either at the hospital or outside it) if you are experiencing any symptoms of depression, anxiety, or another mood disorder (see pages 205–223).

THIS IS NOT YOUR FAULT

As is the case with many issues related to motherhood, it is common for NICU moms to worry that they are somehow to blame for their child needing medical support. That's an understandable feeling, but it is not based in fact. "Prematurity does not discriminate. Every age, every ethnicity, every income level is represented in the NICU," says Kelley. "You didn't do anything wrong. Don't blame yourself," says Kelley. Talking with a peer mentor, the hospital social worker, or another mental health professional can help you internalize that message.

YOU WILL PROBABLY EXPERIENCE SOME
OF THE STAGES OF GRIEF

Whatever the reason your baby is in the NICU and for however long your child is there, it is likely a big change from how you expected to experience the first days, weeks, or months of your baby's life. And that is a loss, says Kelley, whose own children were born sixteen weeks and six weeks early. With her first son's birth, Kelley says, "I lost four months of pregnancy and watching my baby grow. I lost the baby shower, and the birth plan, my husband being there telling me to push, and the celebration of my family coming to meet the baby."

YOU CAN STILL CELEBRATE THE MILESTONES
OF YOUR BABY

There are things you can do to reclaim some of what you have lost and to maintain a sense of normalcy during your stay. "It's important to celebrate milestones during your NICU stay—such as the first bottle or bath—to find and treasure moments of joy," says Kelley. There are also baby books specifically geared toward NICU stays.

RELY ON YOUR COMMUNITY

"This is a time when you call on friends, your community, your coworkers," says Kelley. "People delivered meals to us for months, someone walked our dog, someone cleaned our house." It can be uncomfortable asking for—or receiving—help, but remember, motherhood is not a singular pursuit. It

is a group imperative. It is how humans are intended to grow
the species. If you need a pep talk about why it is not only okay
but absolutely normal and good that you ask for help, read or
revisit page 101.

TAKE BREAKS

Getting away from the NICU regularly is especially helpful
when your baby has an extended stay. "I remember the first
time my doctor suggested that I leave and have a meal outside
the hospital, I thought he was crazy," says Kelley. "But you do
have to sleep, you need to eat nutritious food, stay hydrated,
and maintain close relationships."

It can feel really hard to leave your baby, but you cannot be
there for him if you are depleted and overwhelmed. When
longer breaks away aren't possible, "just walk outside the hospital," advises Kelley. "Moderate exercise such as a brisk walk
and fresh air often help rejuvenate and refresh you after spending hours sitting in the NICU, and then you are going to be
better able to care for your baby."

SET UP A COMMUNICATION SYSTEM

Everyone is going to want to know how you and your baby
are doing, but you have enough to handle taking care of your
baby, yourself, and your family. You don't have time to be a
spokesperson, picking up the phone and answering texts
all the time. Instead, Kelley suggests designating a friend or
family member to post updates to social media or maintain a
blog or other place where you can share the news you want to

share with the people you care about without saying the same thing thirty-seven times.

TAKE CARE OF YOUR EMOTIONAL HEALTH
WHEN YOUR BABY IS HOME

The adjustment at home can be as hard as, if not harder than, your time in the NICU, especially if your baby requires monitoring and you no longer have the experts at your disposal. Make sure you have a good communication system with your provider and keep asking for support and help from family and friends.

"While the NICU stays of my children were the most difficult times of my life," says Kelley, "I can now look back and see so many blessings. I encourage parents to journal, take lots of photos, and find ways to celebrate every milestone, and I also encourage them to seek support from friends, family, hospital staff, and peer mentors. You are not alone. There is an expansive NICU community of graduate families here to support you every step of the way."

Been There, Done That: Moms Talk About the NICU

No books ever addressed how to deal with the NICU. I really felt lost in how to deal with everything. I could not help with his care initially and felt like I was in the way when I was in the NICU and guilty as all hell when I wasn't there, like I was a horrible mom abandoning my baby. For nine days, I could only touch his tiny hand and head, nothing else. Just finally being able to hold him was an experience in bonding. For all the stories about immediate touch and breastfeeding to bond, my son and I did just fine having to wait.   —Nicole, West Virginia

Our son was in the NICU for five days. We didn't really understand what was going on; my partner was so tired but still pumping, and we were afraid he was going to die. The nurses were amazing, and the longer we were there, the longer we got a handle on what was going on with him and what we needed to do to get him out of there. It was still really scary to leave, because I became accustomed to all the machines telling me if everything was okay and having experts close by.   —Donna, Decatur, Georgia

Find at least one person other than your spouse to whom you can go to any time of day or night for anything. I would also highly recommend finding one (or several) nurses to talk about anything, both medically and personally. Seeing them often when you go in to see your child will help the days pass faster as well as put your mind at ease because a "friend" is staying with your child when you can't be there. Take time to take care of yourself. Give yourself permission to be away from the hospital for a bit every day to regroup.
—Amelia, Austin, Texas

At Home: Rest and Rely on Your Village

We used to do a better job of supporting new moms in those overwhelming early days. Back when America was a group of colonies, it was understood that women would need significant time to recover from the physical strain of childbirth and that helping them do so was a community responsibility. Moms were expected to have a "lying-in" period of three or more weeks, during which they would stay in bed, rest, and get to know their babies while family members and other female members of the community brought them food and helped with household chores and infant care. That was the era of "social childbirth," according to *Lying-In: A History of Childbirth in America* by Richard and Dorothy Wertz, a tradition of female community support that was abandoned as hospitals and medical professionals took over the work of delivering children.

But not so in other countries. Today, all over the world, societies follow some kind of postpartum recovery ritual in which little is expected of a mom (often she is expected to stay in bed and be waited on), and much is given to her (meals, massage, even hair washing), all intended to help her heal.

Some are just practices within families and communities, and others are more formalized, like home visits from health-care providers provided by the government. But all of them create an environment in which it is recognized that what you are going through is a really big deal and you deserve support—*a lot of it*—to recover.

Can you imagine if this kind of postpartum recovery period were standard *not only for moms who had given birth but for any family that had welcomed a new baby?* If it were understood that for the next month all you needed to do was meet your baby's basic needs (nutrition, shelter, safety) with help from others and look after your own (nutrition, sleep, physical recovery) with help from others and that everyone else should do the rest?

If that were the case, you would not be feeling pressured to put this book down and clean the dishes before your sister-in-law shows up. You would not feel guilty asking your partner to handle the night feedings. You would not think you were failing at motherhood because the first few weeks felt like a struggle. But so many women do, and that's because as a society we do not send the message that you should be cared for during this challenging transition.

"When I had my baby, a woman gave me a book about a village where the babies never cry, because they are always being tended to by someone in the village," says Kate Lynch Bieger, PhD, a psychologist in New York City who specializes in perinatal mental health and parenting. "And my takeaway was that by myself at home, I should be re-creating this experience that thirty people in a village create. I was always carrying my baby, always nursing, always responding to every need and trying to keep him from crying. It was awful."

It's also completely wrong, as Bieger now readily admits. We cannot do it all by ourselves, and the failure to realize this lies in our societal structures and cultural expectations.

Having help and support is the way nature intended for us to make human beings. Read that sentence again and again and again until you believe it. Then start asking for (and saying "yes" to) help.

A Completely Inadequate Starter List of What Friends and Family Can Do for You Right Now

- Pick up groceries / diapers / wipes, and so on (and maybe just leave them on the porch?)
- Bring or make dinner (if you haven't already, ask a friend to set up a meal schedule through Mealtrain .com or Takethemameal.com)
- Fold laundry (or, better yet, *do* the laundry)
- Sweep and straighten the house
- Make your bed
- Be with the baby (and other children) while you take a shower, go for a walk, take a nap
- Give you a back rub
- Walk the dog
- Take any older children out for a few hours
- Take out the trash
- Mow the lawn
- Wash the dishes
- Pitch in with others to pay for a cleaning service visit
- Run errands with or without you
- Drive you to errands and appointments

Been There, Done That: Moms Talk About Getting Support After Getting Home

Next time, I think I will know better what the average visitor is capable of doing with relatively little instruction, and I would consider making a list on the chalkboard in the kitchen. If they want to help, "Well, there's the list!"

—Jamie, Atlanta, Georgia

Whatever you need, ask for it, because you are worth it.

—Amber, Indianapolis, Indiana

Don't be afraid to be up front with people and say, "It would be a great help if you can do the laundry / do the dishes / cook and entertain my toddler." If they can't handle helping, they aren't the people you want visiting.

—Natalie, Houston, Texas

Don't expect others to anticipate your needs. Ask them nicely for what you need from them. Good friends and family are always prepared to help if you just let them know!   —Anne, Atlanta, Georgia

Korean Americans have it different from Koreans in Korea. In Korea, moms can go to these spa-like centers where you can rest and someone will help you with the baby. For Korean Americans, there's a really different attitude where you're supposed to bounce right back into life.

—Phyllis, Boston, Massachusetts

I did not have a family support system, so I had to hire a part-time helper since I was having a very difficult post-partum period. My mom inferred that I was weak and just needed to "suck it up and deal with it," but hiring additional help was absolutely the best thing for us.

—JENNIFER, ATLANTA, GEORGIA

I definitely find it hard to ask for help in general. I wanted to be everything for everyone all the time. News flash: you burn out. I would recommend establishing your "village" as soon as possible! Whether it is family, friends, neighbors, or random strangers recruited from the street, you need these people. They need you.   —BERNADETTE, MICHIGAN

Your Breastfeeding Survival Guide

reastfeeding is natural." That's a phrase you've probably heard a thousand times by now, and it's true. Women have been feeding babies with their bodies ever since there were women and there were babies. *But* that does not mean it is easy (it also doesn't mean that's the *only* way to feed a baby, but more about that on page 165). Breastfeeding is, in fact, a learned skill. You—and your baby—will have a learning curve, maybe a little one, maybe a medium one, maybe a big one.

"Sometimes it takes a little bit before mothers and babies get the hang of it," says Kathy Kendall-Tackett, PhD, a health psychologist and internationally board-certified lactation consultant (and all-around breastfeeding and maternal mental health expert) in Austin, Texas.

Don't expect to have a home run your first time at bat. It's going to take practice, and you may hit many foul balls. You may get hit in the head by one, and it's possible you could strike out. And I may have taken this metaphor too far. Here's a game plan (sorry, couldn't help myself) for your early days of breastfeeding.

GET SUPPORT AFTER BIRTH

"Take advantage of the free help you get in the hospital as much as you can," recommends Ayelet Kaznelson, IBCLC, a lactation consultant in New York City. "Whether there is someone who comes to your room or you go to a class. Getting good information while you are in the hospital can make a big difference."

Go to as many classes or ask for as many visits from the lactation consultant as possible. Even if you are just receiving positive reinforcement, those visits will help you feel confident when you leave. And, if you are having difficulty, you can ask all your questions, show them what's happening, and get hands-on help to make changes. If the support in the hospital is not available for any reason, you can also call in an outside consultant to visit you (more about how to find one on page 115).

LINE UP HELP FOR HOME

Reach out to a local lactation consultant or breastfeeding class near your home. See page 115 for tips on finding them. If the person you are working with is not supportive of you and your efforts or is making you feel worse emotionally, look for another. It's important that you feel heard and understood.

WHEN IN DOUBT, REACH OUT

There are all kinds of reasons why the beginning of breastfeeding can be bumpy, so "don't be afraid to reach out and ask questions," says Kendall-Tackett. "It doesn't mean you are doing anything wrong, but it's easy to get hung up thinking you are. Even if you just need someone to tell you that you are doing a good job, you can reach out and ask for someone to talk to you about that."

At the "first sign of trouble," Kaznelson recommends "lining up some support, so you can address it as soon as possible. The sooner you address any issues, the less serious they will become."

EXPECT UPS AND DOWNS

"Nursing can be a bit of a roller-coaster ride," says Carrie Bruno, IBCLC and founder of the Mama Coach in Calgary, Canada. "One feed, you think, *I got this; we're good*, and the next feed, you will think, *I'm starving him; why won't he nurse?*"

Bruno also likes to prepare women for an intense feeding frenzy that may hit on day two. "Women often do well in the first twenty-four hours after birth, because they are kind of running on adrenaline, and then quite often on night two, it's physiological for babies to want to nurse and nurse and seem like they are never satisfied. They are wired to do that to help Mom's milk come in. I like to prepare women for that, because that is often when the crash and burn comes in. I find that informing them of that is key."

BUT ALSO EXPECT IT TO GET EASIER

"The first few weeks can be overwhelming," acknowledges Kaznelson. "You are sleep deprived and waking for frequent and long feedings and worrying about whether your baby is getting enough and so on. But that investment pays off later, because it becomes so much easier. The adjustment period is relatively brief—although intense—and that doesn't just go for breastfeeding."

Overall, "you should see an upward trend. Within two weeks, quite often you will feel good about it. Your baby is getting food. You're not hurting, and we would say breast-feeding is 'established,'" says Bruno. "That's the average." But an average is just that; your experience may fall outside of that. That's okay, but if it is feeling very hard, not improving with professional help, and affecting your emotional experience as a mom, you may want to consider reevaluating how you are feeding your child.

DON'T PUNISH YOURSELF IF IT DOESN'T GET EASIER

You have other options. Continue to "If Breastfeeding Is a Struggle," page 165, to read about them.

. . . .
Definitely Get Help Right Away If:
. . . .

- **It hurts.** "Don't grin and bear it," says Bruno. "There will be some tenderness involved, because we haven't used our nipples this way before. But if it hurts, reach out for help right away."
- **Thinking about breastfeeding makes you anxious, upset, or causes dread.** "If there is anything that is not sitting well with you, contact someone," says Kaznelson. "Maybe you just need some

reassurance from someone on the phone, run your experience by someone."

- **Your baby doesn't seem settled after feedings.** "A newborn who is feeding effectively will feed frequently (every two to three hours is average), then settle into sleep until she starts to cue that she is hungry again," says Bruno. "If your baby won't stop crying and does not seem settled, reach out for help to make sure she is getting the calories she needs."

- **Your baby won't wake for feedings.** "All newborns are at risk for jaundice," says Bruno. "If your baby won't wake to feed, it could be a sign she is jaundiced, so bring her into your pediatrician right away."

- **Your baby is not gaining weight or doing so too slowly.** One advantage to meeting with a lactation consultant in person or at a class/clinic is that they can weigh your baby before and after a feed and make sure he or she is getting enough. If your pediatrician expresses concern about your baby's weight gain and suggests supplementation, meeting with a lactation consultant can help you come up with a plan to do so and to improve feedings.

- **Your baby is showing signs of jaundice,** a yellow tint to the skin or eyes, or not waking to feed.

- **Your baby has fewer wet diapers.** For instance, dry diapers for longer than a six-hour period.

- **Your baby shows signs of hypoglycemia,** such

as a low body temperature, shaky hands, a blue tint to their skin, high-pitched inconsolable crying, or seizures.

Been There, Done That: Moms Talk About the Beginning of Breastfeeding

---

The first time, I really wasn't doing it right, despite the help of a midwife at the hospital, and I was in pain for the first few months. It took going to some La Leche League International meetings to get it right. We just need to know how to get the proper support, and that usually means having someone after you are home really be there to watch what you're doing and give advice.

—ELIZABETH, ATLANTA, GEORGIA

I wish someone had prepared me for the possibility of my milk not coming in. I had no idea it could be delayed. I also didn't know I could be supplementing with formula or donor milk, and my baby's weight dropped dangerously. I would have supplemented much sooner if I'd known. We went on to breastfeed exclusively for nine full months.

—LAURA, NEW YORK, NEW YORK

Breastfeeding was hard at first because of blisters, but once those resolved—and it was a brutal week or so—it got much easier.   —JAMIE, ATLANTA, GEORGIA

I had no idea breastfeeding would be so challenging in the beginning! Having support from friends in my new mom

support group helped, as did seeing lactation consultants. You don't just pop your kid on your boob and live happily ever after. It takes patience and a whole lot of practice.

—Amanda, Atlanta, Georgia

If Breastfeeding Is a Struggle

For all the good things about breastfeeding, there are also times when it can be excruciating, not possible for various physical reasons, a real emotional struggle, or something you discover you just plain don't like, and trying to continue begins to have a far greater cost to you or your child than any real or potential benefit. If that happens, you are not alone, and it's worth considering whether you want to continue or switch to formula-feeding or do some combination of the two that eases the pressure on you.

PUT YOUR EMOTIONAL HEALTH FIRST

This is key and something so few of us do. After all, the job of motherhood is to take care of someone else, and usually that's priority number one. But you know what? Taking care of your emotional health *is* taking care of your baby. Feeling more comfortable, not in pain, not preoccupied with stress around how many ounces your baby is getting, or whatever struggles you are facing will make for a much more enjoyable time for you and your baby.

Suzanne Barston had intended to exclusively breastfeed her first child—but a slew of problems, including complications during pregnancy, a tongue tie, jaundice, her son's inability to latch, and postpartum depression made breastfeeding an all-consuming and eventually futile endeavor. The experience was so traumatic and transformational for her that she went on to become a certified lactation counselor and one of the country's leading voices on supporting the feeding choices of all mothers.

"A lot of people can have a lot of difficulty breastfeeding and still feel okay emotionally," says Barston. "But if you are at a point where you cannot connect with your baby, you're not able to function, it doesn't matter if you think you can hold on for another three weeks. You are at a breaking point, and you need to take care of yourself."

When lactation consultant Carrie Bruno meets with moms who are having serious breastfeeding difficulties, she tells them, "You look like you're struggling. You've given it 1,000 percent effort, but this is sucking the life out of you, you're not able to enjoy your baby. It's okay to give him the bottle.' That's usually the moment they've been waiting for," says Bruno.

My hope is that you will give yourself space and permission to figure out the best feeding plan for you *before* you reach your breaking point. But no matter what, it is never too late to take care of yourself.

TALK IT THROUGH WITH SOMEONE YOU TRUST

"When women are sleep deprived, it can be really hard to make these kinds of decisions," says Karen Kleiman, LCSW, founder and director of the Postpartum Stress Center in Rosemont, Pennsylvania. "If you are having breastfeeding difficulties—whether it's supply, your nipples, fatigue—you really need to have a conversation with someone you feel is on your side to help you make a good decision for you. Sometimes the best thing I can do for women is to give them permission to stop." Find your least opinionated friend / family member / acquaintance or a mental health professional and share what you are feeling and ask that they listen and talk it through with you.

CONSIDER SUPPLEMENTATION

If breastfeeding around the clock or pumping and breastfeeding is causing more problems than it is solving, then a first option can be supplementing rather than stopping completely. "It's not always black or white and doing one or the other," says Bruno. "When women are having difficulty, I will say, 'You know we can do both. You can continue to nurse him and top him off with a bottle. There's an array of options.' It's whatever works for that family." And, says Bruno, opting for the bottle at times "does not mean it's the end of your breastfeeding journey. It can be a rest, and that's when you get help."

Work with an internationally board-certified lactation consultant at your home or in a clinic to decide if a combination of formula-feeding and breastfeeding would help alleviate whatever struggles you are facing and come up with a plan to do that.

YOUR CHILD WILL BE OKAY—MORE THAN OKAY

"No matter what, your baby is going to be okay," says Barston. "To me, it's the same as going into birth. Ideally, many of us want to have a drug-free, vaginal birth, but sometimes things don't go the way you hoped and you end up with a C-section. It's not what you intended, but things happen. It doesn't mean you won't have feelings about it, but your self-worth can't be tied to biological functions. And as long as everyone is healthy, it's all okay."

And that means emotionally healthy. That's the goal here. "Millions of babies are raised on formula," says Barston. "I know for a fact what it is like to have postpartum depression and not bond with your child. So the second time around, my priority was that I get that gift and my baby gets that gift. In our case, a present, emotionally healthy mom was more important than breast milk."

"I always say to moms who are struggling, 'What do *you* want?'" says Bruno. "Your baby will be fine however you choose to feed him. I truly believe that. You need to have the energy to enjoy these moments with him. My oldest boy is nine, and now my biggest stress with him is screen time. Nobody asks me at the playground, 'Was he breastfed?'"

IF YOU DECIDE TO WEAN, DO SO GRADUALLY IF POSSIBLE

Find a lactation consultant who is supportive of your choice to stop breastfeeding and, if possible, come up with a plan to wean so that you don't experience the extreme physical discomfort or possible physical and emotional complications that can come with stopping abruptly.

"The more abruptly a woman weans, the more likely it is to trigger some mood instability," says Kleiman. "So, the recommendation is always longer, slower. The more likely you are to protect your mental health." Although she points out that "some people stop abruptly and have no problems."

GET GOOD SUPPORT—GET RID OF BAD SUPPORT

"Make sure the people around you are supportive and shut out the people who aren't," says Barston, who discovered her "Mommy and Me" classes (where everyone was breastfeeding) made her feel worse. "I felt very isolated and angry during those classes, and it wasn't a healthy place for me to be." Barston recommends taking a break from settings that focus on breastfeeding (you can consider going back when you feel more hormonally and emotionally settled with your new feeding plan). Then reach out to online and other communities (see page 366) that are supportive of your choice and feel helpful. "That can be really comforting," says Barston.

CONSIDER BEING THE DESIGNATED FEEDER

One of the great things about feeding with bottles (whether it is pumped breast milk or formula) is that anyone can feed the baby, but if you are mourning the loss of the breastfeeding relationship, "it can help to be the only one feeding the baby," says Barston. "And that's totally okay."

HAVE YOUR "BACK POCKET" RESPONSES

"People are going to ask whether you are breastfeeding, and most of the time they don't mean anything by it," says Barston. In fact, they may be struggling too, but because there is so much pressure around breastfeeding, the question alone can feel like judgment—especially when you are in that fragile, sleep-deprived, post-birth state. Barston found that having some responses ready, such as "Formula-feeding was right for us" helped put an end to painful conversations.

Being ready for intrusive questions when you're in a fragile state is just good emotional self-defense, but the bottom line is that you don't owe anyone an answer. "You don't ever have to give someone—your doctor, a friend, your mother, a stranger—a reason *ever*," says Barston.

If you do switch to formula, see page 118 for tips on bottle-feeding your baby.

If Breastfeeding Makes You Feel Temporarily Terrible—Dysphoric Milk Ejection Reflex (D-MER)

Some women experience a rare but disturbing condition in which they feel profound sadness or other negative emotions right before their milk lets down and for a few minutes afterward. Though it is not well understood, experts say it is a physiological response to breastfeeding.

"It's a hormonal anomaly of the milk ejection reflex that causes an inappropriate reaction of the neurotransmitter dopamine," says Alia Macrina, an internationally board-certified lactation consultant and creator of D-MER.org. "And it causes an intense, but brief, moment of emotional disruption and dysphoria." (*Dysphoria* is a fancy term for "a feeling of unease").

In mild cases of D-MER, one common way women describe the feeling is "like the pang of homesickness you got in your stomach when you were a kid," says Macrina. Moderate or severe D-MER can include feelings of anxiety, panic, and despair or, rarely, thoughts of harming yourself.

Because the feeling often begins even before the tingling of the letdown kicks in, women don't always connect the feeling to breastfeeding and wonder if they are experiencing postpartum depression. The difference, says Macrina, is that D-MER comes on suddenly and eases almost as quickly as it begins. "One minute you feel like, *Oh my god, the world is going to end*, and the next you think, *Oh, the world is great again*," says Macrina, who experienced the condition ten years ago while breastfeeding her daughter.

"When women stumble across the description of the condition," says Macrina, "they usually have an aha moment." And, she adds, understanding the condition is usually enough "to help them feel better and learn how to ride it out." However, she recommends that anyone who experiences D-MER talk with her health-care provider.

Note: Anytime you are having thoughts of harming yourself, contact a mental health professional or the National Suicide Prevention Lifeline to get support right away: 800-273-8255.

Been There, Done That: Moms Talk About Real Breast-feeding Struggles

Making the decision to switch was guilt-filled and awful. At one point, I told my husband that if he uttered the words breast is best *one more time, he was sleeping on the couch!* Fed *is best! My formula-fed babies are happy, healthy, and thriving, and switching was the best decision for them and my family.* —Natalie, Houston, Texas

I remember opening the formula container and just crying hysterically thinking I was such a failure. I was embarrassed and jealous when I saw other moms breastfeeding. Looking back, I was a huge stress ball, and my baby was stressed. I was able to finally take a breath when I started formula, and he was so much better, content, gaining great weight. Don't give up right away, but if you are too stressed, it is okay to say, "You know, this is not right for us." Both my boys were mainly formula-fed. They are smart, sassy, and absolutely beautiful!
            —Stephanie, Traverse City, Michigan

A fed baby is the best baby. A less-stressed mom is the best mom. If you are struggling nursing and stressed out, give it your best shot. If it still is not working, seriously consider either exclusive pumping or formula.
                        —Amy, Houston, Texas

Once we made the switch to formula, our lives became much easier. My little girl was no longer screaming constantly

because she was hungry and irritated. I was still able to bond with her, and her dad had the opportunity to bond with her even quicker. We were able to take turns with feeding, and I didn't have to do all of the work by myself. It was 100 percent the best decision for our family.

—Jennifer, Atlanta, Georgia

I was so overwhelmed and consumed by feeding that I found it difficult to enjoy her. After I switched to formula, I was able to relax a bit. I can't relate when people list enhanced bonding as a benefit of breastfeeding over formula-feeding. While giving my babies their bottles, I can cradle them and look into their eyes, whisper to them, sing lullabies, and I don't have the stress of worrying about things like milk production, latch difficulties, pumping when I am away.

—Amy, Tallahassee, Florida

How to Get Sleep When You Have a Baby

Okay, I'll confess, this section of the book intimidated me. I mean, trying to help moms get sleep when they have a new baby would, on its face, appear to be an impossible task. But, but, but—and this is a big *but*—sleep is so critical to your mental well-being that you and I have to do everything we can to try to help you get more of it. So I'll do my part if you will do yours. You in?

THE CONNECTION BETWEEN SLEEP AND MOOD DISORDERS

"For some women, sleep deprivation is associated with significantly worsening mood and often more anxiety," says Samantha Meltzer-Brody, MD, director of the perinatal psychiatry program at the UNC Center for Women's Mood Disorders in Chapel Hill, North Carolina. "If you've ever battled depression or anxiety at some point—which is a good chunk of women—you need to be mindful of getting enough sleep. The same goes for women who say, 'Yeah, I need my sleep. If I don't sleep, I feel terrible.'"

"Sleep deprivation is not a badge of honor," says Jill Krause, the straight-talking mom behind the popular blog *Baby Rabies*, who experienced both postpartum anxiety and OCD after the birth of each of her four children. "It can trigger a lot of scary things. For me, it triggers bad anxiety, which means I am useless to the entire family. You have to come up with a plan of how you are going to protect your sleep."

BETTER SLEEP = BETTER PARENTING

"Parents spend so much time educating themselves about everything they can do so that their children have the best possible experience, but you can't be this amazing parent if you are exhausted," says Janet Krone Kennedy, PhD, author of *The Good Sleeper: The Essential Guide to Sleep for Your Baby (and You)*. "You don't have the patience or the mood stability. You're irritable. Everything feels like a challenge. You lose the insulation around your nerves, and it feels like your nerves are on the outside of your body."

SHARE NIGHTTIME DUTIES EQUALLY

If you are parenting with a partner, he or she should absolutely be doing as much of the nighttime care as you are. "One of the things I have heard from women is that when they had help available to them during the night from their partners, they felt guilty accessing it," says sleep specialist Leslie Swanson, PhD. "They had this sense they could do it all, and that's just not true. It's impossible. Women's bodies have gone through the biggest changes they will ever go through in the postpartum period, and they need to recover."

"It's really important to advocate for yourself," says Kennedy. "Maybe the other partner has to get up and go to work, but if you are home with an infant, that's hard work too."

Splitting nighttime duties is a little more straightforward if you are bottle-feeding, but there are plenty of ways breast-feeding moms can plan for uninterrupted sleep. For instance, "pump right before you go to bed and then have your partner give your baby a bottle of expressed milk so that you can at least sleep through one feeding," says Kennedy. As the baby grows older and no longer needs to feed at every waking, the non-nursing parent can more easily handle the soothing back to sleep, because, says Kennedy, "if the baby smells breast milk, she's going to want to feed."

GET OUTSIDE HELP AT NIGHT

Another way to get an uninterrupted block of sleep at night, which is especially critical for solo moms, is to have a friend or family member take on some night shifts. Or consider hiring a night nurse (a professional caregiver who will come to your house and handle infant care overnight). Now, before you tell me there's no way that fits in your budget, see a quote from my childhood friend MeiMei in "Been There, Done That" on page 178. She has twins and put night nurse sessions on her registry. Best piece of advice in this book? You decide.

QUALITY MATTERS MORE THAN QUANTITY

By sharing nighttime duties, you can guarantee that you and your partner will get good blocks of uninterrupted sleep, which are so critical to your mental health and energy. Aim, at a minimum, for three-hour chunks. That will enable you to go through an entire sleep cycle and get to the deeper, restorative time of sleep.

KEEP YOUR EXPECTATIONS OF YOURSELF (AND YOUR PARTNER) LOW

"Recognize there are deficits that come along with sleep deprivation," says Robyn Stremler, RN, a sleep researcher and associate professor at the University of Toronto. "Your brain is not going to be working as well as it does when you are well rested. You can't modulate your emotions as well." This ties into the idea of giving your partner the benefit of the doubt (see page 270) when it comes to conflict in this sleep-deprived, non-optimal phase of your life together.

WHEN IT'S NOT WORKING, REEVALUATE YOUR ROUTINE

If you find yourself dysfunctional from sleep deprivation, take a look at the big picture of your current routine and see what needs to change. Try going to bed earlier or sleeping later. "If you feed the baby, she's down to sleep at 8:00, and you're tired," says Stremler. "There's no reason you can't go to sleep then. If you feed the baby at 6:00 A.M., he goes down, and you feel like you could still sleep, then go back to bed."

Been There, Done That: Moms Share Real Stories About Sleep Deprivation and What Helped

With a newborn waking around the clock, I had to rely on my husband to take over for a bit so I could rest. We had a pretty good routine where he would come home from work and take the baby on a walk so I could get an hour or so nap. —AMANDA, ATLANTA, GEORGIA

Hubs and I would break the night into two shifts. I would get up with her 10:00 P.M.–2:00 A.M., and he would get up with her 2:00 A.M.–6:00 A.M. That way, we would each get four hours of "rest" a night. We would rotate each night too, because we knew the second shift was the toughest. —ERIN, DETROIT, MICHIGAN

You know that saying "Sleep when baby sleeps"? Do it. Always. —TIFFANY, HOUSTON, TEXAS

I put night nurse sessions on my baby registry and would recommend other moms do the same, especially if you're older or know you can't deal without sleep. We hired a night nurse to come three nights a week. I couldn't have survived preemie twins without her. Getting three to four hours of uninterrupted sleep, then pumping, then going back to bed for another three hours or so was a godsend. Having a night nurse is way more valuable than just about any "stuff" you could need, other than car seats! —MEIMEI, HONOLULU, HAWAII

I hate the notion that a stay-at-home mom should always be the one to get up while a working father sleeps. I work just as hard every day as he does, and he knows that, so he gets up too.   —NATALIE, HOUSTON, TEXAS

My husband got up every night with our baby, even if he just brought her to me so I could feed her, then he went back to sleep since he was working. So at least I didn't feel like it was all up to me. We always went to bed early (like 9:00 or 10:00) and got up two to three times in that twelve hours, but it was manageable.   —MEGAN, DECATUR, GEORGIA

If someone offers to stay over so you can sleep at night or take a nap, for God's sake, take them up on it!
            —SHELLEY, ATLANTA, GEORGIA

If Your Delivery Didn't Go as Planned

Two-thirds of women report feeling very positive about their birth experience and the care they received. Of course, that means that one-third do not. If you find yourself among the 30 percent of women for whom birth was a disappointment or even a traumatic event, you are not alone. And there are concrete things you can do to come to some kind of peace with the way your baby entered the world.

ALLOW YOURSELF TO FEEL ALL YOUR EMOTIONS

There will be a lot of pressure from friends, relatives, and even medical professionals to put your birth behind you and just be grateful that "you're healthy and your baby is healthy." But there's a big problem with that well-intentioned approach. "That's not the way emotions work," says psychotherapist Sarah Best, LCSW. "If you try to wish them away, or stuff them down inside you, they just come out later in less helpful ways." Acknowledging your emotions is one of the best things you can do.

Some of the Emotions You May Be Feeling
- Sadness
- Anger
- Shame
- Grief
- Numbness
- Disappointment
- Guilt
- Embarrassment

"The first thing you should do is really give yourself permission to feel whatever you are feeling," says Best. "You can love your baby and love motherhood and appreciate that the day your baby was born was a wonderful day and concurrently hate that day and feel upset about it."

TALK ABOUT IT WITH SUPPORTIVE PEOPLE

All the experts on recovering from difficult or traumatic births emphasize the importance of talking about your experience with someone you trust.

One of the most powerful interviews I did for this book was with Pam England, CNM, author of *Ancient Map for Modern Birth*. England launched a new phase of her career as a childbirth educator after her first delivery—which was supposed to be a non-medicated home birth—ended up in the last thing she wanted: a C-section. She now runs a program called Birth Story Medicine in which trained "birth listeners" listen to women share their stories and help them process those stories and come to a deeper, more nuanced understanding of what went down.

Often England says that women begin the process with a belief about themselves, such as "I am weak, because I needed an epidural." England's goal is to help women achieve a more complex and less self-critical understanding of what happened. So that, at the end of a session, a woman might go from "I failed at birth because I had an epidural" to "I didn't like having an epidural, but it doesn't mean I am weak as a person. It was really hard. I did my best."

"A woman can always wish she didn't have an epidural; that's fine," says England. "But wishing she didn't have one is different from believing that she is a bad person because she had one."

HAVE A RESPONSE READY FOR EVERYONE ELSE

"When someone who is well-intentioned or ill-informed tells moms to 'get over it' or 'it doesn't matter,' it's helpful to have a succinct but clear statement in your pocket ready to go," says Best. Something like, "I'm really happy I have this baby, but birth didn't go the way I wanted it to. I'm making sense of those feelings, but I don't want to talk about it right now.' Or 'And I'd like you to listen to me while I talk them through.'"

This may be especially true if you were part of a birth class that had a particular childbirth goal—such as a non-medicated birth. "Some moms who have traumatic or disappointing birth experiences worry about 'When I go back to the class, people are going to ask me how it went.' I recommend they come up with something in advance that they feel comfortable sharing, like, 'There were some complications, and we had to deviate from our plan.'"

KNOW THAT YOUR FEELINGS CAN CHANGE

"How you feel about your birth in the immediate postpartum period doesn't predict how you will feel about it one year, five years, or ten years down the road," says Best. And there are lots of professionals out there like England and Best who can help you find your way to feeling at greater peace (or even positive about) what happened. (See page 367 for tips on finding mental health professionals and England's website, Birthingfromwithin.com, to find a birth listener.)

GET MORE INFORMATION

"Sometimes women who have had a challenging birth experience have a lot of questions about what happened," says Best. "So talking to their care provider or even getting a copy of their records can be helpful."

Best did this when she was considering a vaginal birth after Cesarean (VBAC), following a traumatic C-section with her first child. "It was so lovely to see the nurse's notes from that first birth: 'Mother coping well, mother coping well,'" says Best. "Turns out I was doing really well until there was a serious emergency and I needed an immediate C-section. I didn't 'fail.' It was like the medical record was talking to me."

THE DIFFERENCE BETWEEN DISAPPOINTMENT AND TRAUMA

When Best talks with a client who went through a difficult delivery, she makes sure to look for any signs that she could be experiencing post-traumatic stress disorder, which can happen after a traumatic birth experience, in particular if you felt concerned for your own life or your baby's life during delivery.

See pages 218–227 for a detailed explanation of PTSD, the symptoms that accompany it, and how to get support and help if you experience them.

Been There, Done That: Moms Talk About How They Felt About Their Deliveries

---

I wish I'd understood that babies just do not follow plans. Planning to birth at home and then needing to transfer to the hospital was very disappointing and traumatic. I was angry that the birth did not go the way I wanted it to, and I think all those sunny birth videos did not help. I felt robbed that my birth was not like that.

—MOLLY, MINNESOTA

My birth plan was thrown out the window with my first child because my doctor wanted to induce labor. Ultimately, a C-section was performed. I was angry and wished I had said no to the induction. It took me years to get over the loss of being able to actually deliver my baby. I felt guilty for my feelings, because I had a healthy baby. It took finding an online community of women with similar experiences to finally let go. —MICHELE, MARYLAND

I was induced because of gestational diabetes. After thirty hours, they decided to do a C-section, and because I had been on antibiotics during labor, my son also had to be in the nursery to get an IV. It felt like being kicked when I was

down. When I had trouble breastfeeding on top of it, I felt like my body had failed at all the things women are meant to do. What helped was realizing that what I went through was traumatic, and telling the story. Allow yourself to feel all these things fully and accept that it sucks and what you went through was really, really difficult.

—ELIZABETH, CLINTON, NEW JERSEY

I had an unexpected C-section, and I gave myself permission to grieve the "perfect birth" and that helped a lot. I didn't feel like I had to "Get over it" or "Be happy that I had a healthy baby." I was grateful and happy, but I was also sad and disappointed, and I allowed myself to feel those feelings simultaneously. It aided in my healing and being able to move past the event. But still, ten years later, it's an important part of the story of my life.

—BETSY, ATLANTA, GEORGIA

Bonding with Babies 101

When you meet your baby for the first time, you are beginning a relationship. For some women, the moment feels like falling in love at first sight. For some, it doesn't, and both are perfectly normal.

"There is this myth and expectation that new mothers will fall madly in love with their newborn the minute they pop out, so many women somehow feel defective if they don't have that immediate bond and spectacular love for this baby," says Margaret Howard, PhD, professor of psychiatry and human behavior and medicine at the Alpert Medical School of Brown University in Providence, Rhode Island. "But any relationship takes a while to develop, so there's no rule about when mothers have to fall in love with their babies. Everybody's circumstance is different."

"We all want instant gratification; the image out there is happy family all bonded together instantly after birth," agrees Dana Rosenbloom, MS Ed, a parenting coach in New York City. "More often than not, that doesn't happen, and you get sort of little pieces of that as time goes by and you get more and more connected."

"Part of the problem is that people think that it is supposed to come naturally," says Rosenbloom, "that there is one way to do it, and that there's an exact science to how you are going to bond." In reality, bonding can happen in many different ways and on different time lines. Here are a few things to do to both encourage—and have patience with—the process.

DO THINGS YOU ENJOY

"Bonding happens very naturally when you are happy," says Rosenbloom. "So do things with your baby that make you happy. If you like to lie on the couch and watch *Law & Order*, do that with your baby beside you. If you enjoy sitting by the water, bring your baby and sit by the water. The great thing about babies is that they are portable." (And they don't know how to work the remote yet.)

DON'T WORRY ABOUT WHAT YOU'RE *NOT* DOING

"There are all of these 'supposed tos,'" says Rosenbloom. "You're supposed to do skin to skin; you're supposed to do tummy time. Wipe all those things away. Obviously, there are things that are important to do for your baby's development that will help set them on the right path, but, particularly in the first three months, it's so much more about being together, feeling good and calm and in a positive space with your baby that is what's going to do it."

BE SEPARATE BUT TOGETHER

"Not only do you not have to spend all your time directly interacting with your baby, you shouldn't," says Rosenbloom. "It's a wonderful thing to put a blanket on the ground, put your baby on it, and let him just experience the world." In fact, Rosenbloom is a big proponent of a child development concept called "play in the presence of."

"There's a lot to be said for your children being near you and you being available and present for them but not necessarily directly engaging with them. If you are enjoying the world and you are close to your baby, your baby is going to feel that as close bonding time."

DON'T WORRY IF YOU DON'T KNOW WHAT TO DO

If your baby is colicky and hard to soothe, if you haven't yet figured out which cry means what, it's okay. "Instinct is more about feeling connected than it is about having the answers," says Rosenbloom. "Mothers who naturally just know how to give a baby a bath or have the insight to know 'My baby's doing this; it must be gas' are few and far between. That kind of intimate understanding naturally evolves. Take away the pressure that it should be instant. It takes time."

YOUR BABY CAN TEACH YOU

"The beginning is learning what your baby needs and what you need and how you two will work together," says Rosenbloom. And that kind of learning requires quiet observation. "Some of the most important bonding and engagement comes from sitting back and watching your baby naturally." That's how you will learn how she gets tired, how she relaxes, what makes her smile, and developing that knowledge is the beginning of bonding with—and understanding—your child.

IF YOU'RE NOT FEELING IT YET, THERE IS *NOT* SOMETHING WRONG WITH YOU

"Some women bond instantly and some don't," says Karen Kleiman, LCSW, founder and director of the Postpartum Stress Center in Rosemont, Pennsylvania. "I've never seen a failure to bond as an issue beyond a mom's anxiety about it. Attachment happens. It's biologic. The best we can do for women who are concerned about it is to help them not be concerned about it."

That said, if you continue to worry about connecting with your baby or how you are feeling, you may feel better with mental health support. (See pages 224–227.)

Been There, Done That: Moms Share Stories of How They Bonded with Their Babies and How Long It Took

---

I was surprised how quickly I felt bonded to Frida considering she came into our home as a foster child. I felt an instant and huge responsibility to protect and keep this little being alive, and that dovetailed with warmth and so much love for her. —KRISTEN, SAN FRANCISCO, CALIFORNIA

I was surprised at how detached I felt from my baby after he was born compared to how attached I felt during the

pregnancy. I thought the attachment would "cross over," but in fact, I had to redevelop my attachment to my son when he was outside my body. —ABBY, DECATUR, GEORGIA

It was immediate for me. I just felt simply complete.
—ANGEL, VIRGINIA

People think, Oh, if she doesn't have an immediate emotional tie something is wrong! *And that's just not true. It's like an arranged marriage. There's a sense of duty first that drives the relationship, and the emotional love grows and sweetens the relationship into something really beautiful.* —SND, ATLANTA, GEORGIA

I felt bonded with both of my babies the second they were born. It felt like a love that I had never experienced.
—CARRIE, ARLINGTON, VIRGINIA

It took until she was about a year to feel bonded. Honestly, we grew up together. She grew up, and I grew up into being the mom I never believed I could be.
—ERIN, DETROIT, MICHIGAN

Managing the "Baby Blues"

There's a pretty darn good chance you will experience the emotional roller coaster known as the "baby blues" sometime in the first few weeks after delivery. That's because "the research shows that up to 85 percent of moms will have them," says Karen Kleiman, LCSW.

The "blues," which are characterized by weepiness, intense highs and lows in your mood, as well as a general feeling of being overwhelmed (hello, new motherhood!), and a very low frustration tolerance or even anger, are caused by the drop in hormones that happens immediately after giving birth. All those hormones, which helped your body do all the challenging things it needed to do to bring a healthy baby into this world, can wreak havoc on your mood when they plummet.

Add in sleep deprivation, the physical experience of childbirth, and the massive life transition of becoming a parent (or adding another child to your family), and it makes perfect sense that the early days of having a baby can feel very, very hard—even overwhelming. Your body will adjust to the hormone changes and your mood will likely stabilize as it does, but there are things you can do now to weather this emotional storm. They are outlined in detail in the coming chapters (because they are helpful habits to maintain your mental health at any time), but I will list them briefly here.

EXPECT TO FEEL EMOTIONAL AND MOODY

"You will have moments when you feel joyful and moments when you are overwhelmed and anxious," explains Kleiman. "And that is okay." In fact, some experts suggest we should change the name to the far-less catchy "postpartum reactivity," because many women just experience more intense reactions to things, and those reactions can also be happiness—not just feeling sad.

ASK FOR (AND ACCEPT) HELP

"Do not let feelings of guilt or inadequacy get in the way of letting people help you," recommends Kleiman. "If people are cleaning or caring for you or taking care of your toddler while you take care of the baby, you will get through it much more easily."

DON'T EXPECT TOO MUCH OF YOURSELF

"Take it easy," says Margaret Howard, PhD. "Have other people feed you. Let other people take care of the baby so you can sleep. Stay in your pajamas if that's comfortable for you. Ease into motherhood." (See page 153 for ways to ask for and receive help.)

PRIORITIZE YOUR WELL-BEING

"The mom's experience in those first few weeks is the most important one," says psychotherapist Sarah Best, LCSW. "You might get messages that tell you otherwise, but I am here to tell you straight: your well-being matters most. Pleasing your in-laws, entertaining the neighbors, or doing the dishes should all be relegated to the back burner."

CONSIDER A "NO ADVICE" RULE

"One thing I hear so much in my practice," says Best, "is that much of the unsolicited advice moms get during the baby blues period hits hard. So I really say it's okay to say, 'We have a "no advice" rule in the house right now' or outsource that job to a partner or friend."

TAKE PAIN SERIOUSLY

"Physical pain—whether we're talking about sore nipples, a C-section incision, tearing from a vaginal birth—makes everything so much harder," says Best. If your pain is getting in the way of you being relatively comfortable, get on the line with your provider and address it.

HYDRATE AND EAT

Dehydration can actually create physical symptoms that feel like anxiety, says Best. And birth and breastfeeding can lead to dehydration. So get a good water bottle and have someone keep it filled and by your side. In addition, stash snacks around the house, ask visitors to bring meals, or order takeout if that's an option. "Everything feels harder when your brain doesn't have the nutrition you need," says Best.

GET BREAKS FROM THE BABY

Even if it's just a five-minute walk outside or a good long nap while someone holds the baby in the other room. Get. Breaks. From. The. Baby.

PRIORITIZE SLEEP AND REST

Sleep is one of the best ways to restore your mental health and physical function. See page 174 for how to get good sleep.

SURROUND YOURSELF WITH PEOPLE WHO MAKE YOU FEEL GOOD

Avoid people who don't.

GIVE YOURSELF PERMISSION TO FALL APART

"Women need kindness after they have babies," says Carrie Bruno, IBCLC. "It's a challenging time when women feel uncertain about themselves and can be pretty mean to themselves."

"Let your house fall apart, let your social plans fall apart, let balls drop," advises Jill Krause. "In a few years, none of that is going to matter. In the here and now, you just have to protect your sanity."

WHAT'S THE DIFFERENCE BETWEEN
THE "BABY BLUES" AND PPD?

As many as 20 percent of women experience perinatal mood and anxiety disorders (PMADs) such as postpartum depression or anxiety, so it's important to know what signs point to the fact that some professional help is what you need to feel better.

The key difference between the baby blues and PMADs (see pages 205–223)—such as postpartum depression—is how long you have been feeling this way and how much it interferes with your ability to function (relatively) normally.

"If your symptoms of distress begin or last longer than two to three weeks after delivery, it is no longer considered to be baby blues," says Kleiman. "And some of the emotions of baby blues can overlap with postpartum depression. For example, all new mothers cry, but if you cry all day, for many days, and are unable to function because you are crying too much, that's different."

It's also important to know that some of the most common symptoms of PMADs—persistent anxiety and rage, for instance—don't resemble the placid, sadness-filled woman you may have seen on the hospital PPD pamphlet you were given. But because that is our conventional understanding of what postpartum depression looks like, many women don't realize what they are going through is a mood or anxiety disorder that can benefit from professional support.

THERE IS NO HARM IN GETTING CHECKED OUT

"There is so much pain we could all avoid," says Katherine Stone, the founder of Postpartumprogress.com, who experienced postpartum obsessive-compulsive disorder (OCD) after the birth of her first child fifteen years ago, "if we reach out sooner and realize that we don't have to white-knuckle through this."

That's right. If you are struggling, you don't have to settle for that. "Anytime you are worried about the way you are feeling or thinking," says Kleiman, "it is time to let someone you trust know how you feel."

So check out pages 205–227 for a detailed explanation of perinatal mood and anxiety disorders, the symptoms that accompany them, and how to get the help you need to feel better.

Been There, Done That: Moms Talk About the "Baby Blues"

I felt the baby blues a few days after we were discharged from the hospital. I kept everything to myself because I thought I sounded needy or would feel less of a mother. My husband was the one to suggest reaching out. He provided links to articles and phone numbers to different doctors. He allowed me to spill all my feelings out. That was the start to alleviating the blues. It's normal to feel the way you do. You're not crazy. You're the perfect mom for your baby.

—Tiffany, Houston, Texas

The first three weeks were the hardest of my life. I was all alone, had no real idea what I was doing, and have such an independent nature that it was really difficult to ask for any help. —Jackie, Seattle, Washington

Immediately after my daughter was born, my mood shifted dramatically and quickly. I was sometimes incredibly overwhelmed and sad. For me, this was exacerbated by isolation—spending long days trapped in the nursery with a helpless, demanding human was harder than I thought it would be. I felt more stable and less alone when in the company of other new moms, even more than when I was in the company of my husband or other friends. Find a tribe. Force a tribe. Go to whomever you need to be with.

—JAMIE, ATLANTA, GEORGIA

I grieved being pregnant. I was in such a hurry to meet our son and be a mom, I hadn't really processed that when he was born I wouldn't be pregnant anymore. I went through a few days of missing feeling his kicks and knowing he was safe.   —AMBER, INDIANAPOLIS, INDIANA

I had the baby blues with both kids. I realized I would not experience their labor again and felt depressed that the first days and hours went by so quickly. I cried a lot for "no reason." I talked a lot to friends and my great midwives and felt better after about two weeks.   —CLAUDIA, GERMANY

Why Did I Just Think That? Scary Thoughts Made Less Scary

Have you ever been waiting on a subway platform and thought, *What if I jumped in front of the train?* Or maybe you were driving down the road and for a brief second had a vision of veering into oncoming traffic. These flashes of weird, unexpected, and often uncharacteristic images and thoughts are pretty much universal according to experts. It's the brain's way of testing things out, identifying dangers, and keeping us safe, and parenthood is no different. In fact, "intrusive thoughts," as they are called, tend to bloom in those early weeks and months of trying to keep a small human alive and well.

"Everybody has unwanted thoughts that go against who they are as a person," says Jonathan Abramowitz, PhD, professor and associate chair in the department of psychology and neuroscience at the University of North Carolina at Chapel Hill. "Our brains are creative, and we wonder about whether we could do certain things or whether certain things could happen. That's just how the brain works. That's part of being human."

Abramowitz is one of the country's foremost experts on

intrusive thoughts and has found that "people especially tend to have these thoughts about things that are important to them." (Hello, babies!) Our new babies are really important to us, and keeping them safe is our most important job. So what do we do? Immediately, and understandably, we start to come up with images of potential dangers. We are on the lookout for anything that could possibly harm them, and, yes, that includes ourselves.

In fact, Abramowitz's research has shown that as many as 91 percent of new moms and 88 percent of new dads experience thoughts of harm coming to their babies.

"I think on some level we are evolutionarily programmed to do this," says Margaret Howard, PhD. "Back in prehistoric times, there were lots of dangers lurking, so I think there's still a little part of our primitive brain that has that element of hypervigilance. What it speaks to is a mother's recognition of the fragility of her new baby and also this primal urge that mothers have to protect and keep their offspring safe."

Of course, that doesn't mean that it might not be really scary or uncomfortable to have these thoughts, and many parents are afraid to share them with anyone, says Karen Kleiman, LCSW, because "they think they're going mad, and that if they tell anybody they are going to have their baby taken away."

DO THESE THOUGHTS MEAN I COULD HARM MY BABY?

A lot of women are scared to share these worries, because of the very rare but very tragic stories we hear in the media about moms hurting their babies or themselves. There is an extremely rare postpartum psychiatric emergency, postpartum psychosis, during which women can be at risk for harming themselves or their babies (see page 219 to learn more about this serious, but treatable, condition). But there is one key differentiating factor between the everyday intrusive thoughts most new moms experience and postpartum psychosis (which affects less than one in one thousand new moms), and that is feeling disturbed by the thoughts.

"There is a continuum of possible thoughts from 'Is my baby getting enough food?' all the way to 'What if I take this knife and do something violent to my baby?'" says Kleiman. "It does not matter where your thoughts fall on that continuum; the scarier thoughts are not worse. What matters is how these thoughts make you feel."

For women who experience postpartum psychosis, *if* they have thoughts about harming themselves or their children, the thoughts usually make sense to them and may feel like the right thing to do for the baby. For instance, a mom may believe she has harmed her child in some irreparable way and ending the child's life may seem—in her psychotic state—like the only way to save him from this perceived harm. (See page 219 for a detailed explanation of this treatable condition that requires immediate medical attention.)

However, the vast majority of women experience intrusive thoughts as weird, abnormal, even disturbing, but they don't make sense to them. Rather, the thoughts feel out of character, shocking, and sometimes profoundly upsetting, and there are things you can do to cope with them. It is also important to know whether your response to them is a sign that you are experiencing an anxiety disorder.

HOW TO MANAGE SCARY THOUGHTS

Trying to will these unwanted thoughts away is not going to work. "If you try not to think about a pink elephant, the first thing you are going to think about is a pink elephant," says Abramowitz. Instead, Abramowitz recommends acknowledging and observing the thoughts. When you let them "come along for the ride," says Abramowitz, you can see they're not what they seem to be and develop a healthy relationship with them. "You learn how to be good at having the thought rather than trying to control the thought," says Abramowitz.

And, says Howard, "these thoughts tend to fade with time." Research shows that these worries tend to ebb and flow and may be more frequent around six weeks after your baby is born but then dissipate over the next month or so.

One way to help alleviate the worry that can accompany these thoughts, says Abramowitz, is just educating families before birth about how common they are. That alone can decrease the likelihood that a parent will develop an anxiety disorder related to them. So maybe this section is helping you feel better. Or maybe it isn't.

WHAT IF I CANNOT STOP THINKING THESE THOUGHTS?

For many people, these thoughts can be a passing cloud that doesn't cast a shadow over everything. For others, they can take on a greater meaning. If your preoccupation with them begins to affect your functioning or how you view yourself as a person or a parent, it could be a sign that you are experiencing an anxiety disorder.

Anxiety can develop if you feel so disturbed by your scary thoughts that you begin to do things to get rid of or neutralize the thoughts. You might repeatedly ask your partner if they think a particular bad thing is going to happen. You might continually check your child for scars or indications that they have been harmed, or replay events in your head to make sure nothing bad has happened. Maybe you are going into your baby's bedroom twenty times a night to check that he is breathing.

"The intent of these behaviors is to control the fear or anxiety," says Abramowitz. "The problem is those behaviors make the thoughts more common." Anxiety and unwanted thoughts work like this: the more you try to suppress them, the more you will have them, and then you may actually alter your behavior to avoid the potential harm.

For instance, if you have a recurring thought about dropping your baby over the railing, you might stop carrying your baby down the stairs and ask that someone else do it. Then, over time, you might see the fact that you are not walking down the stairs with your baby as protective for your child. *She is safe because I am no longer carrying her down the stairs.*

If any of this is happening for you, it does not mean you are a bad mom. It does not mean you are a bad person. It does not mean that you are going to harm your child, but what it might mean is that you are experiencing a level of anxiety that is uncomfortable at best and completely debilitating at worst. You deserve to feel better. And, with appropriate treatment, you will.

See pages 205–227 for a detailed explanation of perinatal mood and anxiety disorders, the symptoms that accompany them, and how to get support and help if you have experienced them.

Been There, Done That: Moms Talk About Scary Thoughts During Early Motherhood

---

I had intrusive thoughts of falling down our wooden stairs while holding the babies and crushing them. These thoughts got pretty graphic and troubling, but I didn't mention them because I thought they were crazy, and if I spoke them out loud, someone would take my babies and have me committed. Other intrusive thoughts: car crashes, falling from changing table or crib, dropping the baby on its head, and also intentionally hurting myself.

—JESSICA, ATLANTA, GEORGIA

I would have thoughts like I would hit his head when walking through a doorway or he would be dropped. I could see it in my head. When he got older, it got better, but I still have random intrusive thoughts like I could hit the knife off the counter accidentally and it could impale the baby, or I could trip while holding the baby.

—AMY, HOUSTON, TEXAS

When mine was a few days old—and we were on hour two of screaming—I had this realization when I had her swaddled, holding her tight and bouncing, I kept thinking that it would be so easy to accidently hold her too tight or to jiggle her too roughly, just out of desperation for the crying to stop. This realization that it would accidently be so easy was terrifying.   —JENNIFER, ATLANTA, GEORGIA

The weight of being this person's way of being alive was incredibly heavy for me. My mind began seeking out some of the most dramatic ways I could fail at that, including tripping and dropping him, hurting him. What if I did? It came from a place of realizing how vulnerable he was and how responsible I was.

                        —JESSICA, MINNEAPOLIS, MINNESOTA

When It Doesn't Feel Right: Perinatal Mood and Anxiety Disorders

You may not feel like reading this section. Or you may be really relieved to find that there is a section of the book that openly—and without judgment—explores all the possible ways women can experience emotional complications during pregnancy or after having a child. However you come to this page, I suggest you continue forward with some curiosity and a willingness to see if it is possible that you could feel better than you feel now.

Nobody has a seamless pregnancy or transition to parenthood. I don't care how put together they look or how happy they seem or how on top of the latest advice on baby care they appear to be. Everyone struggles with this wonderful and tectonic emotional, hormonal, and biological shift.

"It's really important to know that everybody goes through a huge transition," says Wendy Davis, PhD, executive director of Postpartum Support International. "That's the natural state of things. There's a whole range of emotions that happen;

some are very temporary and biological, and some go deeper or last longer. That's when we start to assess for a perinatal mood disorder or emotional complications."

MOOD DISORDERS CAN HAPPEN TO ANYONE

Perinatal mood and anxiety disorders (PMADs) are one of the most common complications of pregnancy and childbirth. Up to 20 percent of women will experience a PMAD in pregnancy or after. That's twice the rate of women who will have gestational diabetes.

"When you see those numbers, it's easy to understand that mental health concerns are a really common part of pregnancy and postpartum," says Samantha Meltzer-Brody, MD, director of the perinatal psychiatry program at the UNC Center for Women's Mood Disorders in Chapel Hill, North Carolina. "It is not something to be ashamed of. People easily talk about failing their glucose tolerance test. We need to do the same thing with mental health. You need to take care of yours so you can enjoy and take care of your baby."

THE THREE MOST IMPORTANT TAKEAWAYS
OF THIS SECTION:

We Are Not Just Talking About Depression
You have most certainly heard of postpartum depression, and most of us have a sense of what we think depression looks like—tears, fatigue, lack of interest in life.

While postpartum depression (PPD) can include those symptoms, it is more likely to include other symptoms we don't associate with it, such as anxiety and intense irritability. "Most women with perinatal depression experience some anxiety symptoms," says Meltzer-Brody. And PPD is just one manifestation of what experts now call *perinatal mood and anxiety disorders* (PMADs). These conditions include a range of symptoms and/or disorders that include anxiety, panic, obsessive-compulsive disorder (OCD), and post-traumatic stress disorder (PTSD) and are often a combination of one or more of them. They can happen both during and after pregnancy.

There is also another disorder—postpartum psychosis—that is often confused with PPD but has a very different set of symptoms. We will talk about all of these in the coming pages.

You Are Not Alone, It's Not Your Fault—This Can Happen to Anyone

If you are experiencing a mood disorder during or after pregnancy or as a new mom, you are most certainly not alone, you are not weak, you are not to blame, and you are not a bad mom (and you are not going to be a bad mom). You are just a person undergoing a massive emotional—and often hormonal and physical—transition, and you may need some professional assistance to navigate through it.

Experts are not sure of the exact causes of PMADs, but they do know that the huge hormonal adjustments that occur during and after pregnancy leave some women more prone to developing them. Underlying genetic vulnerability or adverse life events can also increase your vulnerability to developing PMADs, and the natural stresses of pregnancy and new parenthood combined with sleep deprivation can add up to the perfect storm for many women. While there are things (completely beyond your control, by the way) that can put you at greater risk for a PMAD, they can happen to any mom—and they happen to a lot of moms.

These Conditions Are Very Treatable—You Can Feel So Much Better

"When I started giving talks about perinatal mood disorders, I titled them 'The Good News About Postpartum Mood Disorders,'" says Teresa Twomey, author of *Understanding Postpartum Psychosis: A Temporary Madness*, who experienced the condition. "That's because there are not many things in life where you can have something go so wrong that is diagnosable, treatable, and from which you can have full recovery fairly quickly."

"Women that have suffered have every reason to believe that with appropriate treatment they will get better and be able to move forward with their lives," says Meltzer-Brody.

I should know. I'm one of them.

WHY I WANTED TO WRITE THIS BOOK

I'm a good mom. I have a career I love. I have fantastic friends and a really awesome husband (okay, I'll stop bragging). I'm probably one of those moms who looks like they have it all together on the outside (overdependence on Spanx leggings, hoodie sweatshirts, and headbands not withstanding).

Right now, I'm fumbling through parenthood and life okay. I am happy more often than I am sad or stressed, although I still get sad, stressed, mad, and more, because I'm human and this is life.

But there was a time when I was struggling. Every. Day. When I threw up before going to work. When I didn't sleep most of the night. When I was convinced that a bug bite on my baby was the beginning of cancer. Those were awful, miserable, scary months, but when I finally got the help I needed, I felt *so* much better, and I wished that I had done it sooner.

I had a medically difficult pregnancy during which I had to take steroids and other medications and regularly undergo tests to see if I had an autoimmune condition (see page 85 for more on that). It continued after my daughter was born, and I began to worry—nearly constantly—that I had developed a mysterious life-threatening medical condition and that my daughter would succumb to some horrible illness as well.

I went to autoimmune specialist after autoimmune specialist chasing vague symptoms I was certain were deadly. I obsessed over every ailment my baby developed. I woke in the middle of the night most nights and stayed awake worrying about every possible threat to our health. I became such a germophobe that I landed a first-person feature in *Shape* magazine discussing my overzealous handwashing and germ protocols (like, um, using Clorox wipes on every page of every board book my husband brought home from the library).

I had always lived with some amount of anxiety (and had some bad separation anxiety as a kid), but this was over the top. Still, it didn't look like depression, and even though I was in psychotherapy, it took me *nine months* to finally realize that I might need to see a psychiatrist and consider medication to quell the overzealous part of my brain that was calculating risk with the intensity of an insurance actuary.

I finally knew I had to get help when I was on a trip to Jamaica for my husband's work and our daughter face-planted off a high hotel bed onto a concrete floor. The hotel doctor assured me she was fine, but that didn't keep me from staying up every night looking for signs of concussion. I finally broke down bawling on the porch of our adobe cottage as rain fell lightly all around us. "I want out! I want out!" I screamed at my husband.

I didn't want out of my life. I wanted out of my head. When we got home, I went to a reproductive psychiatrist who diagnosed me with anxiety and started me on a low dose of the antidepressant sertraline (Zoloft).

Two weeks later, I felt like a new person. As I wrote in a feature on postpartum anxiety for *Cookie* magazine, "For the overworked alarm clock in my brain, Zoloft is like a permanent snooze button, and I am finally rested."

That was ten years ago, and awareness of PMADs has increased since then, but there are still many women who experience symptoms like severe anxiety in pregnancy or new motherhood and think it's just the new normal. Guess what? It isn't. And with treatment—whether therapy, medication, or a combination of the two—you can feel better sooner than you might think.

So take a look at these pages, see if something resonates with you, and, if it does, keep reading to figure out how you can start feeling better.

ANSWERS TO SOME COMMON QUESTIONS:

Do Women with Postpartum Depression Hurt Their Babies?

It is extremely rare that a mother hurts her child intentionally, but when it does happen, the story is all over the media, which usually (and erroneously) reports that the mom had postpartum depression. In fact, in the very rare instances where a woman harms herself or her baby, she is likely suffering from a psychiatric emergency called postpartum psychosis (see page 219). Like postpartum depression, this is a treatable mental disorder that can occur after childbirth, but they are not the same condition.

How Does PPD Differ from the Baby Blues?

"The fundamental differentiation between the blues and postpartum depression is the timing," says Karen Kleiman, LCSW. "If your symptoms develop after (or last longer than) two to three weeks after delivery, it is no longer considered the baby blues." Also, the intensity of what you are feeling and how often you are feeling it make a difference. "It's not what you are feeling, necessarily," says Kleiman. "It's how often you feel it, how long you have been feeling this way, and how much it impedes your functioning." (See page 191 for more about the baby blues.)

Isn't Anxiety in New Motherhood Normal?

Absolutely. In fact, if you haven't read it already, check out page 198 where I talk about the very normal "scary thoughts" new parents have about harm coming to their babies. Our job as parents is to take care of these new humans, and that requires us to think through the possible threats to their health and safety that we can mitigate. So, of course, you are going to worry about things, wonder if you are doing things right, and call your pediatrician in a panic about something that is totally benign.

But, similar to the difference between the baby blues and postpartum depression, the difference between an acceptable level of anxiety and an anxiety disorder really has to do with how intense your anxiety is and whether it makes it difficult for you to function normally.

What Are the Symptoms of PMADs?

"Most women who experience a perinatal mood or anxiety disorder present with a constellation of symptoms," says Meltzer-Brody. You may feel a combination of depression and anxiety, or you may experience some symptoms of panic or obsessive-compulsive disorder (OCD). Take a look at the list of symptoms below; if you are feeling any of these, it could mean that you are experiencing a perinatal mood or anxiety disorder and will feel so much better with treatment.

- Feeling weepy or overwhelmed for two weeks or more after delivery
- Being unable to sleep even though you are exhausted
- Wanting to sleep all the time
- Crying continuously
- Experiencing constant, intrusive fears or worries (see page 198) that cause you significant distress

- Performing repetitive behaviors or rituals (such as handwashing or checking on your baby) to try to control the worries in your head
- Not wanting to be with (or avoiding being with) your baby because you are afraid of harming her
- Being unable to leave your baby with anyone else or have him out of your sight for fear of him being hurt
- Feeling like your mind is racing with thoughts and you want a break from them
- Experiencing a constant sense of dread like something bad is about to happen
- Having a dramatic change in your appetite or weight
- Worrying that you are going crazy
- Persistently feeling that you have made a mistake by having a child
- Being unable to take care of your day-to-day needs or function relatively normally
- Feeling that your symptoms are unbearable
- Being unable to enjoy your baby at all, not wanting to spend time with her or feeling afraid of her
- Feeling intense rage or constant irritability
- Feeling numb
- Having panic attacks (see page 217)
- Feeling that you have "gone away" or lost yourself
- Feeling hopeless or that things will never get better
- Thinking about harming yourself
- Believing your family would be better off without you or that you never should have become a mother
- Deep down, knowing that something is not right

Experiencing any of these could mean you are suffering from a PMAD and will feel so much better with help. "Any time you are worried about the way you are feeling or thinking, it is time to let someone you trust know how you feel," says Kleiman.

If You Are, Know That:
- You are not alone.
- It is not your fault.
- It makes sense that you are having a really difficult time.
- There are lots of good treatment options to help you feel better.
- You deserve to feel better.
- It is time to reach out for help (see page 224).

What Increases Your Risk for PMADs?
- A personal history of depression or anxiety (in this pregnancy, a prior pregnancy, or in your lifetime)
- A family history of depression or anxiety (in pregnancy or not)
- Having experienced a medically complicated pregnancy
- Having a baby who needed to spend time in the NICU or is having medical complications after birth
- Having a "fussy" baby
- Being a first-time mom
- Not having enough social support
- Experiencing other stresses, such as poverty or financial problems or a job loss in the family

- Having survived sexual assault or other abuse or trauma
- Having had a "high-risk" or medically complicated pregnancy

Often, says Meltzer-Brody, "women who experience panic attacks or OCD in the postpartum period have had these conditions in a subclinical way before pregnancy." That means you may have had milder symptoms of anxiety or OCD but were still able to function normally. Then, says Meltzer-Brody, when you add in the natural (and evolutionarily programmed) tendency toward hypervigilance in the postpartum period, those symptoms can rise to the level of a disorder for which you will need treatment. That was definitely true for me.

Obsessive-Compulsive Disorder

OCD involves repetitive, intrusive thoughts ("scary thoughts," see page 198), and fears that cause you significant distress (such as my concern that the steroids I took during pregnancy had harmed my daughter's immune system). Sometimes you develop compulsive behaviors that feel like they are protecting you from the worry, such as washing your hands repetitively, checking on your baby throughout the night to make sure she is breathing, or, in the case of one woman I interviewed for this book, constantly counting and recounting her supply of pumped breast milk in the freezer to make sure she had "enough."

The research shows that as many as 9 percent of women experience OCD in the first year postpartum.

What If I Am Scared That Someone Will Take My Baby Away?

Many women who are having obsessive, intrusive thoughts keep them to themselves for fear they will be seen as a threat to their child and possibly even have their child taken away.

In the very rare instances in which women harm themselves or their babies in the postpartum period, they are most likely experiencing the psychiatric emergency postpartum psychosis (see page 219), in which they experience a break from reality and thoughts about harming their baby make sense to them. By contrast, women with anxiety are concerned or disturbed by thoughts of harming their baby.

Shivonne Odom, LPC, founder of Akoma Counseling Concepts in Washington, DC, advises moms who are worried about losing their children to reach out to "a correctly trained mental health professional who will understand that you are not a threat to your child and that you need professional mental health support." (See page 370 to find them.) And bring this book with you. Explain the difference in the thoughts you are having—that they disturb you and you are coming to them for help because you want to take care of yourself and your baby.

If thoughts about hurting yourself or your baby make sense to you, or if someone you love is having these thoughts, please read page 219 to learn what postpartum psychosis is and how to get immediate treatment for it.

Panic Attacks and Panic Disorder

Panic attacks are a finite period of feeling intense fear or discomfort when there is no real danger to you. They include symptoms such as:

- heart palpitations
- sweating
- trembling or shaking
- shortness of breath
- chest pain
- nausea
- dizziness
- light-headedness
- fear of losing control or "going crazy"
- feeling disconnected from your body or like you're in a dream

You may feel as if you are having a heart attack or experiencing another life-threatening condition, even though you are physically safe. Experts diagnose someone with panic disorder if she is experiencing repeated panic attacks, constantly worrying that she could have another attack, or if she changes her behavior to avoid the potential of an attack. In other words, if you are having repeated panic attacks or the fear of them is affecting your quality of life, it's likely you are experiencing panic disorder.

. . . .

Post-Traumatic Stress Disorder

. . . .

We usually hear the term *PTSD* in the context of veterans of war, but you can experience PTSD after living through or witnessing any kind of life-threatening event, near life-threatening event or a perceived life-threatening event (in other words, no one's life was actually in danger, but it felt to the person like it was).

When it comes to pregnancy and the postpartum period, PTSD is usually triggered by one of two things: a traumatic birth experience or a history of trauma or PTSD that is triggered again by pregnancy, childbirth, or motherhood. Additionally, parents whose babies spend time in the NICU are at a higher risk for PTSD (see page 145).

You Might Be Experiencing PTSD If You:

- Have a history of trauma and are reexperiencing some of the sensations or feelings related to it
- Had a delivery in which your life or your baby's life was endangered or that felt traumatic to you and you are reexperiencing the sights, sounds, or sensations of your delivery in a negative way
- Feel numb or shut down emotionally
- Are having extreme mood swings
- Cannot sleep even though you are exhausted
- Feel very anxious and agitated
- Are avoiding things that remind you of your childbirth or previous trauma

What Is Postpartum Psychosis?

Postpartum psychosis is an extremely rare (one in one thousand women will experience it after delivery) psychiatric emergency that requires immediate medical treatment. Psychosis means losing touch with reality and is sometimes accompanied by delusions (believing things that aren't true) or hallucinations (seeing, hearing, or feeling things that aren't there). Very often, the disorder will show up in the first two weeks after delivery.

A Woman May Be Experiencing Postpartum Psychosis If She Is Experiencing One or More of the Following:

- Hallucinations or delusions
- Paranoia or erratic behavior
- Extreme confusion
- Euphoria (a weirdly good mood) or mania (being extremely active and productive in a way you would not expect from a woman who is exhausted from having a new baby)
- Doesn't need sleep or is unable to sleep despite exhaustion
- Is having extreme and rapid mood fluctuations
- Cannot put words together correctly, express herself understandably, or is unable to make sense of printed text
- Is insistent that something is seriously wrong with her baby or that she has somehow harmed her baby when all evidence and experts confirm the baby is fine
- Feels like a force is taking over
- Has a compulsion to hurt the baby or herself and believes doing so makes sense or is the right or loving thing to do

"Trust your gut," says Teresa Twomey, author of *Understanding Postpartum Psychosis: A Temporary Madness*, who experienced the condition herself. "If you think there is something very wrong, there probably is, and it is worth seeing a qualified professional to find out what. It might be postpartum psychosis, but it may be anxiety."

Get Help Right Now

Postpartum psychosis represents a real danger to a woman's well-being and the well-being of her baby. Even if women with psychosis are not having thoughts of harming their babies, they are not functioning in reality and are at risk for neglecting their children or putting them (or themselves or others) at risk in other ways.

"You have to get a mom experiencing postpartum psychosis to an emergency room," says Judy Greene, MD, founding director of the Bellevue Hospital's Women's Mental Health Program in Manhattan. "And she will likely need to be psychiatrically hospitalized. Most psychiatric units can treat women with postpartum psychosis."

When you arrive at the hospital, "family members should stay with the mom as much as possible," says Twomey, "for her emotional well-being and for the safety of herself and those around her. If you cannot stay with her, request that she not be left alone until she is admitted to the psychiatric ward or a mother-baby unit set up for psychiatric emergencies."

"If you were having a heart attack, you would not go to work, you would not try to take care of your children, you would get expert medical care to save your life," says Twomey. "And that is what women with postpartum psychosis need. It is not a mental or moral failing. It is a medical crisis that needs medical care."

The vast majority of women who are treated for postpartum psychosis don't hurt anybody and go on to lead productive, normal lives, according to Vivian Burt, MD, a pioneer in the field of reproductive psychology and codirector of the Women's Life Center at the Resnick Neuropsychiatric Hospital at UCLA. "I have seen so many women who have had postpartum psychosis who are wonderful mothers. It is a frightening condition, no question, but when it is properly treated, more often than not, women emerge from it and do beautifully."

See Resources, on page 372, for places to find support and community around postpartum psychosis.

TREATMENT WORKS

All the symptoms and conditions in this section are treatable. Getting help is vitally important for you and your family. Treatment can take a number of forms, including individual psychotherapy, group therapy, medication, or a combination, and there are medications that can be used during pregnancy and breastfeeding. What matters most is that you reach out for help and find a provider who has experience treating perinatal mental health issues or is willing to consult with a provider who does and who offers evidence-based treatment for the symptoms you are experiencing. Go to page 224 to learn how and where to get help.

When Dad Feels Off

I'm writing this book for women, but the mental health of men is also hugely important to the health of families and is largely overlooked. And maybe this book will inspire someone to write a book for dads. In the meantime, here are just a few key things to know:

- Just like moms, dads are going through a massive life transition that involves hormonal, biochemical, and neurological changes as well as emotional challenges.
- Just like moms, dads are susceptible to mood disorders after a baby is born.
- Just like moms, men can feel as if no other fathers are struggling, when, in fact, many are.
- If his partner is experiencing a mood disorder, a dad has an increased chance of developing one himself.
- Recent research estimates that 14 percent of dads in the United States experience paternal postnatal depression (PPND).
- Some research suggests men tend to develop mood disorders a little later than women—three to six months after delivery.
- Our society's ideas about masculinity make it hard for men to admit they are struggling.
- Men are less likely to report emotional symptoms, such as sadness or crying, because of the pressure to appear "masculine."
- Instead, men may exhibit symptoms such as hypersexualization, external aggression, or substance abuse.

- Fathers can find help through many of the same resources I have listed for moms (see page 370), but there are also specific resources for dads (see page 365).

How to Get Help So You Can Start Feeling Better

HOW DO I KNOW IF I NEED HELP?

"You should have a very low threshold for getting help," says Samantha Meltzer-Brody, MD. The first thing you can do is review the symptoms list on pages 212–213. If any of those feelings ring true for you—or if you just don't feel like yourself and know, deep down, something is wrong—then it is time to reach out for support. And if you (or your loved one) are experiencing any of the symptoms of postpartum psychosis (see page 212), it's time to seek immediate medical help.

"Asking for help doesn't necessarily mean you have a PMAD; it means you need help," says Ruta Nonacs, MD, staff psychiatrist at the Center for Women's Mental Health at Massachusetts General Hospital. "There is postpartum illness, but there is also postpartum adjustment, and we want to connect any woman who needs help with their OB, a new moms' group, a psychotherapist. We want them to enter the world of help earlier. If it does turn out to be a PMAD, we want women to know there are different treatments that are very effective, and we want them to be connecting with professionals who have expertise in this area."

THE TIME IS NOW

Many of the experts I spoke to said it was not uncommon for them to see women nine months after a baby was born only to learn that the symptoms started two weeks after delivery. There are two problems with that. One: you've been feeling bad when you didn't have to and you could be enjoying motherhood so much more and so much earlier. Two: the sooner you get treatment, the faster you will be well.

"Getting help sooner is always better than waiting until you are miserable," says Meltzer-Brody. "Research shows that the earlier women are treated for PMADs, the faster their recovery and the less chance they will have a recurrence down the road."

I don't want to lay too heavy a trip on you right now (because I know you are already worrying about so much), but it is also so much better for your child if you feel better. Research shows that when moms are struggling with an untreated mental health disorder, their children suffer too. They are at greater risk for emotional, cognitive, and behavioral problems as they get older. So when women are treated effectively and feel better as moms, their kids are healthier and emotionally stronger. Win-win.

"Look, here's what I want to say to women," says Graeme Seabrook, an internationally certified life coach in Charleston, South Carolina, who experienced anxiety and PTSD after the birth of her first child. "All the things you're worried about right now? When you get help, all those things can get turned around. You can fix all the things that you're scared of."

It is never too late to take care of your mental health. If you have arrived at this paragraph and, like me, you waited nine months (or more) to get help, don't beat yourself up about it. I'm glad you're here. And you have your answer. Now is the time for you to start feeling better.

Where Do I Go to Get Professional Help?

- Your OB or midwife
- Your primary care provider
- Your pediatrician
- Postpartum Support International's Warmline at 800-944-4773. Trained volunteers who have experienced a PMAD themselves will connect you to a provider or support group in your area. You can leave a message that will be returned within twenty-four hours.
- The Seleni Institute, 212-939-7200, www.seleni.org
- The Postpartum Stress Center, 610-525-7527, www.postpartumstress.com, info@postpartumstress.com
- National Alliance on Mental Illness Helpline, 800-950-6264
- Your employee assistance program (EAP) at work

For a detailed list of providers who specialize in reproductive mental health as well as organizations where you can find therapists who treat specific conditions, see page 370.

Note: If you are having thoughts of harming yourself or your child, go to your nearest emergency room or call the National Suicide Prevention Helpline at 800-273-8255.

HOW DO YOU KNOW I WILL FEEL BETTER?

"I very frequently tell my patients that I can say with high certainty they will get back to their baseline level of functioning. It may take weeks, it may take months, in some cases it may take a year, but you will get there," says Judy Greene, MD. "One of the things that drew me to this subspecialty is that the outcomes are really great."

The recovery time frame varies depending on the condition you are experiencing and how long you have been experiencing symptoms, but many women start to feel significantly better in a shorter period of time than they expected.

"It is a real trial by fire," says Katherine Stone, the founder of Postpartumprogress.com. "But one thing you take out of it is a sense of what you are capable of and how you are capable of finding tools to take care of yourself. That's important. Knowing that you can endure something terrible, seek help, and that you can get through it."

And when you do, you will be in really good company (if I do say so, myself): the company of women who have fought hard to feel better, improve their lives, and improve the lives of their children and families.

How Can I Tell My Family and Friends That I Am Struggling?

Ideally, for all of us, there is at least one person in our lives with whom we feel comfortable sharing all our feelings, even the hard ones. If you have that person in your life, start there. If you don't, pick the person who you feel is most open-minded or best able to work well under pressure—someone who you think will listen and then take action and help you. If you can't think of who that person might be (or you just don't want to talk to someone you know personally), then get on the horn to the Postpartum Support International Warmline (800-944-4773). (See a complete list of resources for getting help and support on page 370.)

Do not stop talking until you find someone who will help you.

The Added Pressure of Infertility or Adoption

Many women report feeling guilt that they worked so hard to become moms and now they aren't able to enjoy being a mom—and people in their lives may reinforce this idea. "You always feel like you can't complain because people say, 'You asked for this,'" says June Bond, executive director of Adoption Advocacy in Spartanburg, South Carolina, who actually coined the term *Post Adoption Depression Syndrome* (PADS) in an article in 1995. PADS is estimated to effect as many moms as perinatal anxiety and depression (see page 368 for emotional support resources for adoptive families). In fact, the struggles of infertility and assisted conception and the stress of the adoption process can actually put women at a greater risk for developing a mood disorder.

Whatever path you took to arrive at this new place in your life, it is understandable if you are struggling. If you find that other people do not understand that, explain to them that just like any other new mom, you are vulnerable to mood disorders at this time of your life. It does not mean you do not love your child or that you don't feel deep gratitude that he is here. It just means you are also struggling and deserve support to feel better.

HOW TO TALK ABOUT IT

Wendy Davis, PhD, encourages women to start the conversation with the basic message: "Lots of women have this, there are a million ways to treat it. I want you to know that I am going through this, and I need your support."

Suggested Conversation Starters

- "I've been having a really hard time, and I need you to listen to me and help me."
- "It turns out that a lot of people have depression and anxiety in pregnancy and after a baby is born. It's way more common than I realized, and I think that is what is happening with me."
- "I'm really concerned about how I have been feeling, and I need help from the people who love me, like you."
- "I've been feeling really badly, and I've learned that what I am going through is not uncommon and there are things I can do to help me feel better, and I need your help."
- "I want you to know what's going on with me and not be afraid to talk to me about it."
- "I've learned that taking care of your mental health is a really important part of having a strong family, and I want to take care of mine now. Will you help me?"

REMEMBER THAT THEY ARE LEARNING TOO

Your family and your community may not have much information about perinatal mood and anxiety disorders. That can be frustrating and a little intimidating, but it is also an opportunity for you to put into words what you have been feeling, what you have learned, and what you need, and that can be a really powerful experience as you work to feel better. And, of course, you can always just hand this book over to them, ask them to read "When It Doesn't Feel Right," and then come back and talk with you!

KNOW THAT WHEN PEOPLE ARE SCARED THEY SOMETIMES SHUT DOWN

Just like a lot of women with PMADs might not want to admit to themselves how bad they are feeling, the people in your life may want to minimize your feelings as a way to protect themselves from their worry about you. That's human nature.

"It's helpful to understand what people's fears are," says Katherine Stone. For instance, if your partner tries to reassure you that you will feel better, and it's not that big of a deal, Stone recommends trying to figure out what he or she is worried about, so you two can talk directly about those concerns.

THINK ABOUT WHAT WILL MOTIVATE THE PEOPLE IN YOUR LIFE TO HELP YOU

Just as it's important to understand the fears that may hold people back from helping you, think about what matters to them and appeal to those issues to elicit their support.

"There will be people—and there are cultures and communities—who don't believe in mental illness or medication for mental health," says Stone. In those cases, you can get folks on board by "helping them think of it as getting parenting support."

If they are opposed to the use of medication, you can open the conversation by explaining that therapy is one of your options.

Some cultures or communities value the well-being of the group over that of the individual. If this is your family's or community's approach, it can be helpful to explain that by helping you as a mom, they will be strengthening your family and, by extension, your community.

Stigma: When Your Friends, Your Family, or Your Community Do Not Understand the Importance of Mental Health

As a society, we are really uncomfortable talking about mental health. I think it's safe to say that many of us are afraid of the topic, and often misinformation informs people's response. That can make it even harder to get help. Here are some things you might hear on your journey to get better.

- "You can pray this away."
- "Snap out of it."
- "You're just too sensitive."
- "Mental health or psychotherapy is for _____." (Fill in the blank)
- "You are too strong to need help."
- "You're being selfish."
- "There's nothing wrong with you."
- "You just have to get through this."
- "Be positive!"
- "This should be a happy time."
- "You must have done something (in a past life or a sin) to make this happen."

- "What did you do to cause this?"
- "We don't talk about our private business outside the home."
- "Don't make our family look bad."
- "You just need to _____." (Fill in the blank: get outside, exercise, eat better, sleep more, try harder, etc.)
- "But you're not crazy! "
- "Therapy is the easy way out."
- "You're just being dramatic. Everything is fine."

Responses like these reflect other people's biases and fears and cultural and community misperceptions around mental health. They are not about you. You are listening to yourself. Don't let them stop you from doing that. Ask them to read this section of the book. Direct them to the resources in the appendix. Keep talking until they listen. If they won't, talk to someone else who will.

Someday, these outdated notions of mental health will truly be a thing of the past, but you don't have time to wait for that. The time to help yourself is now.

IF ALL ELSE FAILS, APPEAL TO THEIR CONCERN FOR YOUR KID

You deserve to feel better and enjoy motherhood and your life, and that is all the reason in the world you need to take care of your mental health. But I also know that the welfare of kids is a big motivator for folks, and if you need to, you can certainly couch this conversation in terms of your child and your family's well-being. Research shows that when moms are struggling with an untreated mental health disorder, their children suffer too. They are at greater risk for emotional, cognitive, and behavioral problems as they get older. So when women are treated effectively and feel better as moms, their kids are healthier and emotionally stronger.

Share that information with the people you need to help you. Or pass the buck to a health-care provider, such as "My pediatrician thinks that it will be better for the baby if I get some professional help to feel better."

Moms of Color

Any mom can develop a perinatal mood or anxiety disorder. However, research into PMAD prevalence shows that moms of color—particularly black and Latina moms—experience PMADs at higher rates than white women and are much less likely to receive treatment for them. Some research suggests that Asian Americans and Pacific Islanders are the least likely to receive mental health care in the United States.

There are a lot of reasons for these disparities, including the fact that a disproportionate number of moms of color experience risk factors for PMADs such as the added stress and trauma of racism and poverty. There is also an appalling lack of providers of color and services offered in communities of color, and a history of mental health care that has been developed by—and for—the white community. All of that needs to change and is slowly, slowly improving.

Another barrier can be stigma and stereotypes specific to a particular community. Of course, the term *moms of color* encompasses so many different moms that there is no way to generalize about what your experience may be if you are a mom of color. Even within specific communities, your experience is your own, but it is possible that, on top of the general stigma about mental health in our society, you will run into some expectations or beliefs within your community that make it difficult to talk about what you are going through. See "Stigma: When Your Friends, Your Family, or Your Community Do Not Understand the Importance of Mental Health" on page 232 and "Think About What Will Motivate the People in Your Life to Help You" on page 231 for some suggestions of how to help them see past their initial ideas about mental health.

Psychotherapist Shivonne Odom, LPC, meets with African American moms weekly who are struggling with the idea of reaching out for support. "We've been socialized that we can get through anything," says Odom. She tells her clients, " 'You are going to be okay. You love your baby. You're a great mom. Everything's not broken inside. Your maternal instincts are intact. You want to get help for you, and that means you are getting help for your kids.' "

There are also mental health issues specific to being a racial minority, including the trauma of discrimination and state-sanctioned violence that deserve knowledgeable and compassionate support.

We know that before anyone can reach out for help or make change, they need to feel heard and understood. For many moms of color, that may mean finding support specific to the community you come from and the challenges you face.

In the appendix (see page 369), I have included organizations, websites, blogs, and books that offer support, resources, and mental health care specific to different populations of moms so that, if you want to, you can seek them out. And know that whatever messages you get from the culture at large or the culture in your living room, you deserve support to feel better and you can find it.

REALIZE IT MIGHT BE HARD FOR PEOPLE TO "GET IT"

Even my very supportive, incredibly open-minded husband could not understand what I was feeling at the height of my postpartum anxiety. "But what you're saying doesn't make rational sense!" he would say to me even as he tried to listen and comprehend what I needed.

"It's very hard to help someone understand something they haven't been through and that they can't see and touch," says Stone. If you find that the people you love can't wrap their brains around what you are saying about how you feel, Stone recommends sticking with a more informational approach. "You have to say, 'These are very clear signs of an illness. It happens to 20 percent of mothers, and if I don't get help for it, it will get worse. In order to avoid that, I need your help.' There are practical arguments you can make that take the emotion out of it."

The other thing both Stone and Davis emphasize is that it is possible not everyone in your community will come around. "It's really important that women not wait for the endorsement of others to get help," says Stone. "In the end, you have to take care of yourself, because you're all you've got." (See "How to Get Help So You Can Start Feeling Better" on page 224). "If someone can't talk about it, it's really okay to step back from that person," says Davis. "Find the people who will be supportive."

And keep talking until you find someone who will help you get the support you need to feel better.

Been There, Done That: Moms Talk About PMADs

I had postpartum anxiety and felt like my brain was constantly racing. I was terrified all the time. I jolted awake constantly to stare at the baby to make sure she was breathing. I literally shook in fear for an hour when my sister and cousin took the baby for a walk in her stroller. It was irrational, constant fear. I didn't know what I was feeling wasn't normal. I didn't talk to anyone.

      —LAURA, NEW YORK, NEW YORK

Once I started to open up to friends, I found many more had it than I ever knew. It's just no one talks about it! It felt so good to know I wasn't alone.

      —ERIN, DETROIT, MICHIGAN

After my second baby, I was so sure that my baby would get sick and even eventually die and that it was some secret only I knew. I had this feeling of impending doom for longer than a year. I also started to feel increasing anger. I had to make getting a good night's sleep a priority—so I night weaned and created a plan to get my children to sleep in their own bed. I also started exercising more, which really improved my mood and helped a lot with patience. Eventually I went on an antidepressant.

—ANONYMOUS

I went through PPD that I never talked about. Instead, I just posted cute baby pictures, so I'm sure the perception was, "You're doing so great at this and you're such a great mom," when inside it's a daily war.

—BRANDY, CHICAGO, ILLINOIS

I talked to two of my good girlfriends and told them I was worried I might have PPD, and they kind of brushed it off like, "No, you're fine. It's totally normal." I know they were trying to be helpful, but it's also totally fine if I did have PPD and needed some help. If a new mom is hesitant to share how she is feeling, I would just say do it!

—AMBER, INDIANAPOLIS, INDIANA

I felt like I could not talk about it. I was a stay-at-home mom when my daughter was first born, and the message was, "You're staying home, you're not even going to work, what could be troubling you? You shouldn't be having any problems." Mental health stigma was definitely part of that, and also in the Korean community, it's just something that nobody ever talks about; as parents, we never talk about the tough parts of parenting.

—PHYLLIS, BOSTON, MASSACHUSETTS

I was extremely open about discussing my PPD and anxiety. Everybody has a hard time. It's perfectly fine to admit it. Talk about it! Your life—and your baby's life—will be so much easier once you start receiving help.

—Jennifer, Atlanta, Georgia

After two miscarriages, I had anxiety and depression during my pregnancy with my son. I still smiled, showered, wore makeup, dressed the part, but inside I was a mess. I wasn't sleeping, constantly felt there was something I needed to be doing, and I couldn't relax to the point I would make myself sick. After a year of this, I went to my regular doctor and described my symptoms (while crying), and she diagnosed me with PTSD/PPA/PPD. I immediately Googled PPA and bawled over the symptoms. It described exactly what I had been going through. I started seeing a therapist and took antidepressants for a year. The therapist saved my life and is one of the best things I've ever done.

—Lisa, Houston, Texas

There is always someone who will help. Keep reaching out until you find that person. Don't give up if you don't feel like yourself. —Anne, Atlanta, Georgia

Taking Care of Your Body Instead of Beating It Up

The idea of "getting your body back" after pregnancy is kind of ridiculous when you think about it. You've grown a person inside—and then pushed them out of—you! This is a massive life transition, and it's way easier to look forward to where you are going than to try to go back to where you came from. For now, that means taking the pressure off focusing on how you look and putting the attention on recovery and how you feel.

"Give yourself a break and understand that it's normal to have a flabby body," says Kate Lynch Bieger, PhD. "Your body did exactly what it was supposed to do, and now you need to take time and rest it instead of getting back to the way you want to look," says Bieger. "Getting out for walks or other exercise is all about giving yourself self-care and nurture to get back to yourself."

START SMALL

"There are so many ways to be active and move your body," says Christina Hibbert, PsyD, author of *8 Keys to Mental*

Health Through Exercise and a clinical psychologist in Flag-staff, Arizona, specializing in maternal mental health. "It doesn't have to be going to the gym; it doesn't have to be for an hour. It can be ten minutes twice a day, three times a week. You don't have to push yourself, and you don't have to overdo it. Maybe it's just 'Today I am going to walk to the mailbox and get the mail. By the end of the week, I will walk to the end of the block. Next week, I will walk around the block.'"

GET OUTSIDE

"A lot of moms struggle with low energy," says Frances Largeman-Roth, RD, nutrition expert and author of *Feed the Belly*. "But if you get outside and feel that sunshine and get that vitamin D, it does wonders for your mood."

TRACK HOW YOU FEEL

Kate Hays, a clinical psychologist in Toronto, Canada (who was pretty inactive until her son was two years old), now incorporates exercise into her treatment with patients. She actually does therapy sessions where she walks or runs with her clients. Isn't that cool? But her advice is not to take it from the experts. Instead, prove the value of exercise to yourself.

"Track your mood. Are you tense? Sad? Whatever you're feeling, rate it on a 1 to 10 scale before you do an activity," recommends Hays. "Write it down in a notebook or put it on your phone." Then do the same thing when you finish moving your body. Very quickly, says Hays, "you will realize (a) you should be doing this for yourself, and that (b) it makes you feel good."

Jotting it down is key, says Hays, because it's likely you will have some epiphanies in the moment that can vanish in the seconds it takes for your baby to cry when you walk in the door or unstrap her from the carrier or stroller. If you notice something different about yourself later in the day, reflect on that too, because the benefits can be unexpected. According to Hays, movement can increase your ability to problem solve effectively. Show me a parent that doesn't need that and I'll pay you a portion of any royalties I (hopefully) get from this book!

REALIZE WHAT YOU ARE CAPABLE OF DOING

"Part of the excitement about being physically active can be discovering, 'Oh, this is what my body really wants to be,'" says Hays. In fact, there is research that shows a "connection between physical strength training and feeling mentally stronger." I can vouch for that with my own experience. When I moved to Atlanta and joined a fitness camp, I became stronger than I have ever been in my life, and that strength made me feel much more capable in all areas.

"From a psychological perspective," says Hays, "exercise can bring a feeling of mastery, like, 'I am really accomplishing something.'" And when you are on the hamster wheel of basic childcare—feeding, diapering, getting to sleep—doing something that feels like it is accomplishing something can be huge.

I'm not saying you aren't accomplishing something monumental when you take care of your child's basic needs—you're nurturing a human; that's huge!—I'm just saying it doesn't always feel like you are, and being able to walk farther or walk faster, run a 5K, lift more weight, or swim five laps without stopping can help you to feel a sense of success you may not be in touch with in other areas of your life.

WAYS TO MOVE YOUR BODY

If physical activity has not been a regular part of your life before now, Hays recommends being "experimental and curious" about what kind of activity you will enjoy and actually want to do. And start slowly. In the beginning, walking (maybe just around your bed initially) is probably all you can manage. Wait until you are fully recovered physically for more rigorous activities. When you are ready, here are some things to try:

- Walking outside (put your baby in the stroller or carrier)
- Window-shopping (put the baby in the stroller or carrier) for ten to twenty minutes
- Yoga (check out community centers and your local YMCA for affordable options with childcare included!)
- Postnatal yoga videos on YouTube (many are just five minutes!)
- Group fitness classes geared toward moms, such as Fit4MOM, Strollercize, Baby Boot Camp, Oh Baby! Fitness, Stroller Warriors (for military moms)
- Cleaning the house for ten to fifteen minutes
- Gardening for ten to fifteen minutes

- Running (stop into your local sports store to find out about local running groups of all levels; my town has one just for moms)
- Dance classes
- Zumba
- Tai chi (often offered at community centers)
- Team sports (moms' softball team, local women's soccer league, grown-up kickball)
- Online workouts, such as yoga through your TV service or on your computer
- Workout DVDs
- Exercise apps (there are lots of quick ones that you can work in at any time)
- MuTu Mama (an online program to help restore your core after that baby did a number on it!)
- Jump on the trampoline with your kids (good luck not peeing your pants!)
- Play tag with your kids

Been There, Done That: Moms Talk About Getting Moving

Walking with my baby in the Ergo was my favorite part of the day in the first year or so. I stayed in shape and lost weight too! —Kristen, San Francisco, California

I was super lucky that I was involved in a program called Stroller Strides, which was a workout where you bring your kid and everyone hung out and got to know each other

after the workouts. That was the best thing I did for the first year of each kid's life.   —KATE, ATLANTA, GEORGIA

I exercised once I was cleared by the doctor around six months. I started off slowly with yoga and slowly got into cardio and weight training. It made me feel so incredibly great, it gave me a little break, and I could clear my head!

—KAITLYNN, MANITOBA, CANADA

I signed up for a mommy/baby yoga class. It wasn't a rigorous workout, but I'm so grateful I did it. I definitely felt like it helped me feel better faster. I remain close friends with almost all the women in that class.

—JAMIE, ATLANTA, GEORGIA

When my son was seven months old, I started doing at-home workouts through an online streaming service. This was perfect for me because I didn't have to be away from my son and could work out when it was convenient.

—AMBER, INDIANAPOLIS, INDIANA

Being a Mom to a "Fussy" Baby

All babies have times when they are "fussy," a.k.a. crying a lot or nonstop. For some babies, this occurs during a particular time of day (usually from about 4:00 to 7:00 P.M.) and for a set period of time (typically two weeks to twelve weeks), but about 10 percent of babies spend most of the time unhappy about something or other. Often these babies are diagnosed with colic or reflux, and there are a number of approaches to and treatments for easing the infant's distress and helping them feel better and cry less. But for many, it's just who they are.

CHECK IN WITH YOUR PROVIDER

Holly Klaassen, author of *The Fussy Baby Survival Guide*, founder of the Fussy Baby Site and the mother of one colicky and one high-needs baby in Vancouver, British Columbia, tells all parents to see their pediatrician with any concerns they have. "The vast majority of the time, a fussy baby has colic or it's his temperament, but if your gut is telling you something is wrong, keep pushing for answers."

Once the tests have been run and the doctor says, "Your baby is perfectly fine," Klaassen says, the next stage is accepting your baby for who he is and finding ways to cope.

ACCEPT AND ADAPT

"A lot of the time, parents drive themselves crazy wondering, 'What did I do to cause this?' 'Why can't I fix it?'" says Klaassen. "I tell them, at a certain point, it's time to adjust your expectations. This is who your baby is. You didn't do anything to cause it. You don't need to do anything to fix it. Now it's just time to adapt. I find that approach often helps parents feel like a big weight has been lifted."

IT'S NOT YOUR FAULT

"When a mom says to me, 'I just don't know what to do. I feel like I am failing at this. I just can't make him happy,'" says psychotherapist Sarah Best, "I emphasize that some babies are just wired this way. Having a good relationship with a pediatrician can help minimize self-doubt." They can help you troubleshoot and reassure you that colic and fussy babies are something that happens and not something you caused.

FEELING ANNOYED AT YOUR BABY IS NORMAL

One of the first things Birdie Meyer, RN, coordinator of the Perinatal Mood Disorders Program at Indiana University Health in Indianapolis, tells moms who live with fussy babies is, "It's really hard to like a baby who cries all the time." And most of the time, when she says that to moms, says Meyer, they end up crying themselves, because "they've thought it."

"Anybody who got screamed at by another human being around the clock would find themselves kind of annoyed," agrees Best. "It doesn't mean you don't love your baby; it just means that being screamed at all day long is really, really hard."

YOU NEED TO PRIORITIZE BASIC SELF-CARE

"Having a fussy baby is going to get under your skin; there's no way around that," says Best. "But it might get under your skin less if you had a sandwich, a chance to pee, or a shower." Basic self-care (which may be all you can do right now) becomes really important. "There are certain things you need to do for yourself to feel human. For instance, showers are a nonnegotiable," says Klaassen. "Put him in the crib or in the bouncy seat and take one."

YOU NEED HELP TO DO SO

If you are raising your baby with a partner, now is the time to really pull together as a team and swap shifts. If you are a solo mom or your partner is not as available as you need, ask friends and family to spell you during the hardest times of day. If it is within your means, hire a night nurse or sitter to be with your baby during the night so you can get a break from screams and get the uninterrupted sleep you will need to manage the days. You can also ask folks to pitch in to a "night nurse fund."

IT'S OKAY TO WALK AWAY

"When a mom is dealing with a really colicky baby that is crying all the time, I insist they get relief," says Kate Lynch Bieger, PhD. Even if you don't have someone helping out, "you can put the baby down in a safe space and you can walk away, close the door, and take a breath."

YOU NEED BIGGER BREAKS FROM THE BABY

"Go for a walk, get a cup of coffee. Even fifteen to thirty minutes to yourself can be game changing," says Best. Many moms report feeling guilty—especially if they enjoy the time away (who wouldn't?!)—but your baby needs a mom who is as mentally healthy and strong as she can be.

Klaassen recommends tag-teaming or recruiting a grandparent or close friend and sleeping in the basement, at a friend's house, or, if you can afford it, in a hotel room for the night. "Your baby will be okay, and it can really recharge you," says Klaassen. "Even if you can only get away once a month."

CONNECT WITH PARENTS WHO "GET IT"

"Forty percent of babies are easygoing," says Klaassen, "so, many of the parents you encounter will have an easy baby and a lot of them will think it's something you are doing." That's why it's critical, says Klaassen to find support among parents who understand what you are going through. "Surrounding yourself with people who are going through the same thing, makes you realize, 'Okay, it's not just me.'" See page 366.

WORK IN TEENY, TINY WAYS TO EASE
YOUR STRESS

"There is time for a little self-care in every moment," says Bieger. She recommends that her clients try out smaller types of self-care like pausing to gently rub on a lotion that smells good to you, breathing in the calming smell, and feeling a kind touch on your skin (yes, yours). "It might feel ridiculous, but giving yourself whatever moment of pleasure or nurturing you can shifts your emotional stability when you walk back into the room."

Other Ways to Center Yourself in Stressful Moments
- Run your hands under warm water
- Take a quick shower
- Sit down and breathe deeply for a few minutes
- Write down a mantra to say in difficult moments ("My baby's okay" or "This time will pass")
- Sing to yourself
- Hug yourself or do other self-compassion exercises (see page 335)

YOU DON'T HAVE TO SOLVE THE PROBLEM

"As parents, you assume that you will always be able to do something to soothe your child," says Klaassen. "Before I had my son, I didn't understand that some babies are unsoothable and it's not our job to stop the crying. Especially when they are newborns, there are times when you just let the crying happen."

When Best talks to moms who are struggling with fussy babies, she likes to share this finding from the literature on attachment: "It's presence and effort that an infant picks up on. Even if you are not always able to soothe your infant (and if she's fussy, that may be rarely), she is really picking up on your effort and presence." In fact, even when your child is crying, research shows that being with you lowers his or her stress response.

Often there is no calming a colicky baby, and it is in those moments that one of the hardest parenting lessons can be learned: "Good parenting isn't necessarily making the pain go away," says Bieger. "It's letting the child know you are there."

THAT WON'T STOP EVERYONE AND THEIR MOTHER FROM THINKING THEY HAVE THE SOLUTION

Once again, good intentions meet total obliviousness when you are out and about with your fussy one and the clerk at the store, grandma in line, or, hey, your mom, offer their tried-and-true methods that you have no doubt already attempted. "When people give you tips, I say just smile and nod," says Klaassen. "Because you can go crazy trying to convince people that you really have tried everything." If you want a back-pocket response ready, here's one: "Thanks for the advice, but the research shows this is just how some babies are born."

THIS TIME WILL PASS

"The vast majority of even the most colicky babies get over it by twelve weeks," says Janet Krone Kennedy, PhD. "It can feel endless, but it is temporary."

To move through it, Kennedy recommends "accepting that this is a very intense and temporary period that you need to get through. It's not an indicator of the kind of baby you have or what the rest of your life will be like. You just have to get through this time."

PROFESSIONAL MENTAL HEALTH
SUPPORT CAN HELP

If you've been dealing with an inconsolable baby, then it might not shock you to learn that having a fussy baby is a risk factor for developing a perinatal mood or anxiety disorder (PMAD) such as postpartum depression or anxiety. In fact, some research shows that having a baby who cries inconsolably can double your risk of experiencing a mood disorder. If you do not feel like yourself, flip to pages 205–223 to read through the symptoms of perinatal mood and anxiety disorders. If you are experiencing one, you can feel so much better with the right kind of support.

Been There, Done That: Moms Share How They Coped with Having a Fussy Baby

---

Our daughter had acid reflux, so the first month was hard. It was very overwhelming at times to not be able to help her feel better, but I continually reminded myself that she was safe and getting the most love possible in my arms.

—Anne, Atlanta, Georgia

My baby has terrible reflux. She cries from 4:00 P.M. to 11:00 P.M. every day. It is hard. I manage it by giving her to my wife and taking a shower every night at around 9:00

or 10:00 so that I can have some quiet and peaceful time to myself.   —ALEXANDRA, ATLANTA, GEORGIA

Getting out, walking, and any kind of motion really helped and was calming to the both of us. I tell parents when you get overwhelmed (not if you get overwhelmed), lay the baby down in a bassinet, swing, anywhere safe, and walk away. Take a break. The baby won't die from crying.
—STEPHANIE, TRAVERSE CITY, MICHIGAN

My daughter was a big-time crier, so when people would visit they would hold her for me so that I could take a small break from the crying. I would do anything to feel normal again: nap, shower, eat, clean, so that I could feel as if I had control of something.   —JENNIFER, ATLANTA, GEORGIA

I felt like a terrible mom. I felt like I failed nature. How could I not fix her? I would put her in an Ergo and play Pandora and dance around the house. In retrospect, I think that helped both of us.   —ERIN, DETROIT, MICHIGAN

Taking Care of Yourself from the Start

I f you gave birth to your baby, you've just come through months of constantly making choices to take care of yourself for the baby inside you. You probably avoided certain foods, added in others, maybe you changed your exercise routine or started one, and tried to lower your stress—all in an effort to give your baby the best environment for healthy development. And, yes, some of those changes may have been difficult, may have made you resentful at times, and might have felt like a burden, but you *did* them. The funny thing about motherhood is that it makes it easier to make sacrifices and to prioritize someone else's well-being.

My great hope for this book is that it will give you permission, encouragement, and the tools to make your well-being as great a priority as that of your child and your family.

TAKE BREAKS FROM THE BABY, AND LET SOMEONE ELSE BE IN CHARGE

"Early on, I recommend that parents develop a certain level of normalcy with being away from the baby," recommends Sheehan David Fisher, PhD, assistant professor of psychiatry and behavioral sciences at the Feinberg School of Medicine in Chicago. If you are the primary person who is home with the baby, then Fisher recommends "getting out of the house for a half hour or more every day. Go to a park, be somewhere scenic. It gives your body an opportunity to regulate itself."

If your partner is available to take care of the baby while you do so, even better, says Fisher. It's an opportunity for him or her to connect with the baby and for you "to mentally let go." In fact, when Kathryn Lee, RN, a sleep specialist in San Francisco, researched ways to help new moms get good sleep, she found that one of the most helpful things the new moms in her study did was write up a contract for the dad (in her study the partners were all men) to leave work an hour early and bring home dinner or be responsible for making it.

"That way, the mom knew for sure that she could get a shower, go for a walk, or whatever she wanted to do and the dad could bond with the baby," says Lee, "and it made all the difference. For at least half of the women in the study, that was what got them through the day. And the dads really enjoyed the bonding time with the baby." Win-win!

If you're a solo mom or you just can't make a schedule like that work, recruit friends, neighbors, or, if it is financially possible, hire a sitter.

IT'S OKAY IF YOUR CHILD'S NEEDS COME AFTER YOURS

"Thinking of yourself first and then the baby is unusual advice for a new mom," says Hara Ntalla, MS Ed, the clinical director of the Seleni Institute (where I serve as editorial director), "but doing so is absolutely necessary. When you recharge, she will recharge. When you give yourself permission to enjoy the small pleasures of life, she will learn to do the same. When you prioritize your well-being, she will do the same for herself."

"The thing that helped me the most as a new parent—which I know is counterintuitive—was taking a break from my baby," says Abigail Marateck, LAMFT, a therapist (and good friend of mine) in Decatur, Georgia. "My sister came to town when my son was a few weeks old. She encouraged me and my husband to get out for a little bit. We went to a local dive bar, and it was the best hour *ever*. I felt some semblance of myself, which I needed to feel. This feeling fueled me even more than sleep. It was like a high five to myself."

MAKE MOM FRIENDS

This is the one piece of advice that almost every expert I talked to gave me. It is critical when you are adjusting to your new life as a mom that you find supportive moms who will listen to—and normalize—your struggles and be good company in what can be a very isolating time. (No offense, infants, but you kinda suck at conversation.) And having good social support is one of the best things you can do to take care of your mental health now and forever, especially because there are going to be times (more than I want to think about) when you will forget to take care of you. And you know who is really useful when that happens? Good friends.

The great thing is that new motherhood is a terrific time to find them. Like starting school or a new job, you've got a pool of people from whom you can pick those that resonate with you.

That's an important point.

At first, I thought that just sharing the bond of motherhood was enough for a friendship to bloom, and I headed down a few dead-end friendship streets with people that were just not right for me (kind of like my early dating life, but I digress). I have met a lot of moms in the decade that I have been a parent, and I have developed deep bonds with only a handful of them. But all the other moms I have met have still been a valuable part of me getting my sea legs as a new mom (even if sometimes I just needed confirmation that the choices I was making were best for me).

I met one of my best mom friends on the playground when she just asked me straight up if I wanted to start having playdates. I knew she was my mom soul mate then, because she was as eager as I was to connect, and she remains one of my closest friends. So keep putting yourself out there until you find your people. If that's hard for you (like I think it is for most of us), think about how someday you are probably going to have to give a shy kindergartner a talk about how hard it can be meet new people, but it's how you make friends. Practice now and you won't feel like a hypocrite when you do! (I told you I was not below stooping to guilting you into taking care of yourself!)

Places to Find Mommy Groups or Meet Other Moms

- Where you delivered
- Local children's stores often coordinate groups by delivery date
- Community centers
- Story times at local libraries and bookstores
- Fitness classes (especially "Mommy and Me")
- Meetup.com
- Facebook or another online community
- Parent support groups (such as PEPS in Seattle)
- MOPS (a nationwide Christian organization that connects moms)
- Your religious organization
- National Healthy Start
- Breastfeeding clinics, classes, and organizations such as La Leche League

. . . .

Find Safe Spaces

. . . .

As with making friends, not all moms' groups are going to feel comfortable and familiar to you. If they are organized around a particular parenting approach that doesn't mesh with yours, you might feel alienated or judged. If you are working in an office and all the moms in the group are staying at home, you may not feel all your experiences are understood or you might just feel lonely. I had a friend who was part of an online moms' group composed of primarily white moms. As a mom of color, she didn't feel understood or safe among a group that she felt didn't understand or even want to understand her experience and concerns as a mom of color.

This is not to say that moms with office jobs and stay-at-home moms or co-sleepers and Ferberizers or moms of different ethnic or racial backgrounds can't be good friends and good support to one another. Of course they can! But what matters is that whoever you are and whatever your approach, experience, and background, you find spaces that feel safe and encouraging to you as well as spaces where your issues will be heard and understood. Move on and look elsewhere if they don't. See page 374.

SMALL MOMENTS OF SELF-CARE

"I focus a lot on micro self-care," says Lori Mihalich-Levin, founder of Mindful Return, an online course for moms heading back to work, and author of *Back to Work After Baby: How to Plan and Navigate a Mindful Return from Maternity Leave.* "Things you can do in a short amount of time."

- Appreciating how good a shower feels, focusing on how good the warm water feels and the fact that you are alone for a few minutes
- Short, guided meditations or breathing exercises on an app or on your own
- Reading (or listening to a book) only for pleasure
- Keeping a nice-smelling lotion on hand to lovingly apply to yourself in moments of high stress

Do everything you can to begin to make self-care a practice from the very beginning of your life as a mom. Put your emotional and physical health at the top of your priorities and practice caring for it in small ways daily, weekly, and monthly. If you can begin your parenting life with this outlook, I guarantee it's going to get easier, more manageable, and more enjoyable. And, when you're ready, you will have the instinct to launch into the bigger forms of self-care (see page 310) that will sustain you throughout motherhood.

Surviving Early Parenthood
as a Couple

Spoiler alert! Most couples have a hard time when they become parents, and though that probably seems like the kind of thing you don't need research to prove, there is research to prove it. "What we know from our research is that about 67 percent of couples—no matter the variables, their socioeconomic status, level of education, or cultural background—struggle," says Joni Parthemer, master trainer of the Gottman Institute's Bringing Home Baby program.

That may not be a happy statistic, but is sure as heck makes sense. For as long as you and your partner have been together, you have been the focus of each other's worlds. Now there's another person who needs attention. A lot of attention. Like, basically, all the attention. Plus, she hasn't learned to sleep through the night yet, so you're both exhausted and operating with very short fuses. And you're learning how to meet her needs, so you're both probably a little anxious. One of you is likely going through a major hormonal shift. Maybe one or both of you is experiencing a mood disorder. Maybe your sister is staying in your house and you haven't been alone in two weeks. And maybe one of you (I'm guessing you if you are the one reading this book?) is staying home with the baby and taking on the lion's share of the baby care. Or maybe you are both leaving the house each day to work and trying to fit everything else in when you get home. I could go on and on.

It makes total sense that in this environment, conflict will find a foothold. At least it did for pretty much all the women I surveyed for this book (see "Been There, Done That") and for me. "Let's be realistic," says Parthemer. "None of us knew how hard it was going to be. No matter what people said to us, becoming parents affects every fiber of our being." Amen, sister.

In the early months of my first daughter's life, I proposed that my husband and I have a joint session with a therapist. I had an agenda: to prove in a neutral setting—with an expert to verify it—that I was doing all the work and deserved all the sympathy and support. I don't know whether the therapist pulled some kind of Jedi mind trick on me, but somewhere in the middle of the session, it became apparent that both my husband and I were working our tails off and we just couldn't see it. I was a little sad to give up my martyrdom but really grateful we had a good place to hash out what we were feeling and what we needed to each feel supported in that super difficult stretch of early parenting.

That was not our only session we've had since becoming parents (and I am sure it will not be our last). Sitting down with a professional, objective observer can help you and your partner find clarity in a very muddy time. It also gives us tools to address the inevitable conflicts that occur. But therapy is expensive, not always covered by insurance (though more and more it is!), time consuming, and not everyone's cup of tea.

So here's a little cheat sheet to making small changes to weather the relationship roller-coaster ride of new parenthood.

HAVE YOUR PARTNER READ THIS SECTION

Maybe the whole book?

GIVE YOURSELF A BREAK

"Conflict comes with the territory of new parenthood, especially when you are sleep deprived," says Sheehan David Fisher, Ph.D. When Fisher works with couples after delivery, he helps them understand that you don't have to see catastrophe in every conflict. "An argument can just be an argument based on what you guys are going through," says Fisher. In other words, no matter how tough this patch gets, don't start spinning doomsday stories in your head. This is a very specific moment in time.

FOCUS ON LITTLE IMPROVEMENTS

You don't have to go on a daylong '80s rom-com montage date complete with kite-flying to stay in touch with your partner. Focusing on the daily ways you interact can make a big difference in keeping connected in the beginning. "People think it's a lot more difficult than it really is," says Parthemer. "If we monitor and adjust in small ways, we can stay on the same trajectory."

And that's where the flip side of the 67 percent of new parents come in. "One-third of couples tend to navigate these stormy seas," says Parthemer. The Gottman Institute analyzed the couples who were doing well to see if the things they did could help couples that were having a harder time. "They did three things," says Parthemer. "They strengthened their friendship, had a soft way of dealing with conflict, and viewed themselves as a team."

SOME WAYS TO DO THAT:

Talk About Things Other Than the Baby

When it's 9:00 P.M. and the baby is finally asleep, don't just turn on the TV and ask each other about logistics—"Did you get the diapers?"—says Fisher. Instead, try to focus on "some of the things that brought you together in the first place" like talking about politics or telling funny stories or listening to music you both love, a little something to remind yourselves of why you started on this mad journey of raising a human being together.

To connect with what the other person is feeling, Parthemer suggests asking open-ended questions. Here are some conversation starters:

- "What was the hardest thing you did today?"
- "Did anything make you laugh today?"
- "How did that presentation you were worried about go?"
- "What did you do during the baby's nap?"
- "Is this whole parenthood thing what you expected so far?"
- "What do you miss about our pre-parenthood life?"
- "What is making you happy right now"?
- "What do you want our life to look like in five years?"

- "What's it like to see me as a mom?"
- "What were some of your all-time favorite dates we've had?"
- "What kinds of dates should we go on when we can?"

"Just having a conversation that feels more normal to you can go a long way to feeling better together," says Fisher. And asking some larger questions about this time together will help you stay in touch with the bigger picture and connected to how you are feeling.

Offer Small Words of Appreciation

"We know that *even* when couples are doing well, when they are together 24-7, they miss 50 percent of the positive things that are going on between them," says Parthemer. That's probably because we are programmed to find and fixate on the negative (so we could keep ourselves safe from danger back in the day). Research from the Gottman Institute shows that you have to express five positive things to your partner for every one negative statement to keep things stable.

Now, when you are sleep deprived, jacked up on hormones, and overwhelmed by the demands of new parenthood, there may be a lot of negative comments flying. But when you can, offer a kind word or a simple "thanks" for the things your partner does for you. If he or she doesn't follow your example, ask them to.

Even If Problems Seem One-Sided, the Solutions Can Be a Team Effort

If your baby is not sleeping as much as you want, if your nipples are cracked and bleeding, if one of you is intensely irritable, do your best (I know you won't always succeed, because you're human) to approach these problems as ones that can be solved together.

No, the non-breastfeeding partner doesn't have the cracked nipples, but he or she can go out and find the ointment that will relieve them or call the lactation consultant. If your partner is irritable (even if he or she is taking it out on you), you can both stop and ask what you can do together to help him or her release the stress in a more positive way. Even if you can only manage to do this a small portion of the time, you'll be learning the valuable lesson that problems can pull you together rather than drive you apart.

Get Away in Manageable Ways When You Can

"You may not be able to go on a weekend getaway," says Fisher, "but you need to get out of the house." Maybe it's a date. Maybe it's getting ice cream for an hour together while the neighbor sits with the sleeping baby. Think about what "you can do together in a short period of time that will give you the biggest connection bang for your buck."

"Every parent we met in the kingdom of parents who bragged they hadn't been to the movies in five years and thought it made them the best parents of all, those were the ones that got divorced," says syndicated sex columnist Dan Savage. "It's the parents who took some time away that are still together. It's not a selfish thing to do, and it's not neglect for your kids to go to Grandma's while you spend time together."

Make a Plan for Both of You to Get Self-Care

This is going to be really challenging in the first days or weeks home, but as soon as you can, identify something you both do that is key to your emotional well-being (see page 314 if you need some ideas). For my husband, time alone with his journal keeps him emotionally grounded, so in the early days of parenthood, he would take his journal to the Laundromat with him. While our copious loads of onesies and spit-up cloths spun in the big commercial machines, he sat across the street in a bakery and wrote in his journal. The laundry got done, and he got his alone time. Win-win.

WAYS TO MANAGE CONFLICT PRODUCTIVELY:

Don't Play the Martyr

That is probably the most hypocritical piece of advice I have given in this book. Because. I. Play. The. Martyr. All. The. Time. Sometimes it makes me feel a little superior, but it never moves the needle of relationship satisfaction, not one bit.

In more emotionally mature moments when I am able to see that my husband is working (almost) as hard as I am and can approach the problem with some compassion and understanding of his struggle (even if I will never believe it is as hard as mine), we get so much further in coming up with solutions together.

Cool Off and Repair

Of course it's normal to feel angry, but you won't get very far solving a conflict if you are so mad all you can do is rage at your partner. It's important that you take a break until one or both of you calms down enough to talk calmly about the issue.

When you return to the conversation, you might want to start with a little repair work. "We are all going to screw up and say mean things we wish we didn't," says Parthemer. "When we do, it's about catching ourselves and saying, 'I need a break' or 'That was below the belt.'"

. . . .
When Anger or Conflict Feel Out of Control
. . . .

If you feel unremitting rage toward your partner, it could be a symptom of a perinatal mood or anxiety disorder that can be treated so you feel better. And if your partner is experiencing anger disproportionate to the conflict, he or she could also be experiencing a mood disorder. See pages 205–223 (and page 222 on paternal postnatal depression) to see if either of you might benefit from professional support to feel better.

And if either of you is resorting to verbal or physical abuse, it is imperative that you get help. See page 363 in the appendix for organizations and hotlines that can connect you to professionals who will help you manage the situation right away and help get your family to safety if necessary.

Begin with How You Feel, Not What Your Partner Is Doing "Wrong"

At the Gottman Institute, "when we videotape couples having conflict," says Parthemer, "we can tell in the first three minutes how it is going to end." How? By the way the disagreement started.

"It's all about how the conflict is brought up," says Parthemer. When conversations start with criticism or contempt or blame, "the conversation usually goes downhill pretty quickly." Instead try a "softened start-up," which means beginning the conversation gently.

Here Are Some Samples and Swaps

- "You hurt me." Try: "I feel hurt by what you did."
- "You never empty the diaper pail." Try: "Would you do a few rounds of the diaper pail emptying? I need a break from the smell."
- "I'm always the one who gets up in the middle of the night." Try: "I'm really wiped by the middle-of-the-night wake-ups; can we come up with a schedule to take turns getting the baby when she cries?"
- "I never get a moment to myself." Try: "I feel like I have not been by myself in days. Could you take the baby while I get out with a friend / take a bath / lie down for a thirty-seven-hour nap?"

It's much more effective to think about (and then express) "what's important to you, what you want the person to understand, and how you want them to help you," says Fisher.

Be Open to How Your Partner Feels

"It is really challenging to hold somebody else's reality in your mind without creating your rebuttal," says Parthemer. "You don't have to agree with it, but you need to be able to communicate back to your spouse what they are feeling and show that you've heard them." Everyone feels more inclined to work through a problem when they feel their concerns are also on the table.

Figure Out Your Nonnegotiables

In her workshops, Parthemer helps couples identify which problems are solvable by creating a diagram. "There's a smaller circle in the middle of a larger circle. At the center (in the smaller circle), put things that you cannot yield on, things that are the core of you." Then in the outer circle, put things you can yield on."

Having an understanding of what those are for each of you will help you both respect the issues that matter most to one another. For instance, my husband couldn't care less if the house is neat, but after years of talking about this issue, he now understands that a neat house is a prerequisite for me to feel calm, and he works to keep it neat because he knows it affects my mental health so much.

Give Each Other the Benefit of the Doubt

This one does not apply in a relationship where one partner is being abusive to, or emotionally controlling of, the other (see page 268). In those circumstances, professional support is what you need (see page 363) to see if your partner can change and your relationship can be a safe space for you and your child.

But assuming your relationship is operating on mutual respect and care, chances are all the things you are doing that drive each other crazy right now are not being done with malicious intent. "By giving your partner the benefit of the doubt, you reduce the natural defensiveness and combativeness that arises when malicious intent is assumed," says Fisher. "This allows you to listen to your partner's opinion and empathize with their perspective even if you don't agree with it." And that's how you get to dialogue, and, ultimately, resolution.

Been There, Done That: Moms Share How They Worked Through Conflict with Their Partners

---

Try, try, try not to compare who has had less sleep or who changed more diapers or whatever. No one wins that contest. —SHELLEY, ATLANTA, GEORGIA

Being honest about how tough it is in the beginning helped; at times we both looked at each other and said, "This sucks." But each hard stage will pass. Take turns as much as you can; you are both in the trenches those first few months, but then it gets better.

—STEPHANIE, TRAVERSE CITY, MICHIGAN

We tried to be extra cognizant of the fact that we weren't sleeping well and that tensions were high, and we tried not to take anything personally. We also had to have many frank discussions on what was going wrong and what we could do to fix it. It took us a good year to get back on track as a couple. —JENNIFER, ATLANTA, GEORGIA

I recommend making an effort to spend some regular time alone together, even if it's just hanging out watching a movie in bed without cell phones on. Ask each other how you are holding up so that you have opportunities to help each other out without the other person having to bring it up.   —ANNE, ATLANTA, GEORGIA

One thing that was really important was keeping up kind acts for each other. I know it sounds insignificant, but it is easy to get wrapped up in the baby's need and neglect one another.   —BERNADETTE, MICHIGAN

We had some marriage counseling that was very helpful.
   —KIMBERLY, DECATUR, GEORGIA

A baby, by necessity, has to be the center of the family for a while since they have so many needs. But at some point, you have to work to keep your relationship strong. It's the foundation of your family, and it'll be what you have left when your kids flee the nest.
   —AMANDA, ATLANTA, GEORGIA

A Low-Key Guide to Sex
in Early Parenthood

.

SCREW THE SIX-WEEK CHECKUP

Most women will see their birth care provider six weeks after delivery to see how things are going down there, and many people (and health-care providers) view this visit as the "sex clearance" checkup. If your vagina or your incision looks sufficiently healed, then you and your partner are free to go about having all the wild sex you have spent the last six weeks daydreaming about. And, to be fair, if you have, and your provider gives you the A-okay, who am I to stand in your way? But on the off chance that getting down is the last thing on your mind right now, I am here to offer some reassuring perspective and baby steps forward.

YOUR BODY MAY NOT REALLY BE READY

"Everyone's recovery is totally different," says Michigan sex therapist Sarah Watson. "Your body has been through the most enormous change in your life. So to only give yourself six weeks to return to your pre-pregnancy sex life is a little unreasonable."

SEX MAY BE THE LAST THING ON YOUR MIND

"At six weeks, you're probably up every two to three hours. You're not taking a shower every day, and you're probably feeling overwhelmed," says Watson. "You may not have had any time to think about feeling sexy, and that's okay, because your whole focus has been keeping this baby alive." Also, if you are breastfeeding, the hormones helping with your milk supply have a dampening effect on your libido. Many of the moms I surveyed said their sex drive did not really come back until after they weaned.

YOU COULD FEEL "TOUCHED OUT"

New babies are so dang cuddly, but they are also *on* you. All. The. Time. If you are breastfeeding, then they are attached to your breasts a good number of their waking hours. All that intimacy can be wonderful and cozy and delicious. It can also be stifling, hot, sweaty, and even claustrophobic at times.

If that's the case, the idea of another human sidling up to you may be unappealing at best or abhorrent at worst. You may feel like you just don't want one more person touching you, which is perfectly understandable.

YOUR BABY MAY BE MEETING YOUR
INTIMACY NEEDS

This is something I often felt in the early years of both of my daughters' lives. I got such satisfaction from cuddling them that I felt very little—really, no—need for intimacy from my husband at times. "You are getting all this dopamine from the baby, and it makes sense that you wouldn't want to get that elsewhere if you are getting it from nursing or cuddling with your baby," says Erin Martinez, a couples' therapist in Dearborn, Michigan, who specializes in sex therapy. (Phew! It's normal!)

I'm lucky that my husband didn't take this personally, even though he wished it were different. But it's understandable if a partner does, says Martinez. "Your partner can feel left out of the process, that they've been replaced or are not needed," says Martinez. "If you are having that sort of sexless feeling, I would remind your partner, 'We decided to do this together, and we're just making it through this time period. It's not forever.'" Then talk about how you want to reconnect as your baby gets older.

SEXUALITY AND MOTHERHOOD MAY NOT SEEM LIKE A MATCH

"Some women feel they are completely mommies now and that they are not sexual people," says Watson. "I usually tell them they need space where you are not being a mommy in order to think about yourself in a sexual way again. Before I even get into talking about date nights, I like to give moms space to be adults, to talk to other adults about adult topics, to enjoy taking care of parts of their body. I think the first haircut you get after having a baby goes a long way to feeling a little bit like, 'I am able to take care of myself.' Giving women the space to do those things before they feel a responsibility to feel hot and sexy."

THINK ABOUT WHAT KIND OF TOUCH (IF ANY) YOU WOULD LIKE

"I encourage women not to feel like it is a 'yes' or 'no' answer to intimacy," says Martinez. "Think about what might feel good to you. What kind of touch you would like. What will help you feel connected, loved, and attractive." Martinez sees this as an easier way to warm up to intimacy again and gives you something to build on in conversation with your partner. "Rather than saying, 'I don't want to do that,' you can say, 'I would love to do this.'"

If you're breastfeeding, "breast play may be off the table for a while," says Watson. "Your breasts are now a source of food and probably not a source of pleasure. Your nipples may be chapped; your breasts may feel engorged." So, if your breasts are a no-fly zone and you're not ready for penetrative sex, think about what you would like and what might feel good to you—a nice light back tickle (one of my faves), massage, oral sex, a hand job?

KEEP IT LOW-STAKES

"If you're too aggressively tending to your sexual connection out of fear, then sex becomes just one more thing you have to do," says Dan Savage, author of the long-running Savage Love column and creator of the *Savage Lovecast*. And we all know the to-do list of new parents is long enough. On the other hand, Savage says, if you are not sustaining some level of sexual connection, it can be hard to get it back.

His solution? "Adjust your expectations of what's possible.

Keep it on a low simmer for a while. Neither my husband nor I had to give birth," says Savage. "But we did have the exhaustion of having an infant in the house and the relay race of that. So we masturbated together for a while. It was a way to keep the flame alive. Our approach was, 'This is all we can do for now, and this is pretty good.'"

REDEFINE "SEX"

If vaginal penetration is your end goal, then there's a pretty good chance one or both of you is going to be disappointed in the weeks and months (year?) following the birth of a baby. But if you can expand your idea of what sex is, it becomes easier to incorporate it into your life more readily (especially because some of the alternatives are much quicker!).

"A hand job is sex, and it can be really great sex," says Savage. "Someone holding you while you masturbate and saying a few dirty things to you is sex." Looked at this way, you can have a pretty active sex life—if you want to—not too far into new parenthood.

See page 82 for a fun list of all the things you can do that don't involve penetration.

JUST DO IT FOR YOURSELF

"Rather than trying to fit into your partner's needs, think about what turns you on and invite him or her into it," says Mara Acel-Green, MSW, psychotherapist and owner of Strong Roots Counseling, a fantastic clinic focused on supporting women and families, in Watertown, Massachusetts (check it out, Boston readers!). "Don't rally for your spouse. Rally for yourself! Get naked, touch yourself a little, then let him do it."

JUST DO IT FOR YOUR PARTNER

"I think the secret to my husband's and my success," says Savage, "is that we didn't wait for the times when we were miraculously horny at the same time. We took care of each other. We called it 'assisted masturbation.' I would help get him off, and the bonus was that sometimes I would get in the mood too. We were recognizing our responsibility to each other erotically and making an investment for the future."

Of course, you should never feel coerced to meet your partner's sexual needs. If you do feel that way, or if you are experiencing any verbal or physical abuse in your relationship, then you need to reach out for some professional support to find your way to a safe relationship or out of an unsafe one (see page 363).

WHEN YOU DO DECIDE TO "DO IT"

"It's going to feel different the first time you have intercourse," says Martinez. And if you have any pain, listen to it. "It might be your body's way of saying, 'I'm not healed enough.'" In that case, Martinez recommends checking in with your doctor to make sure everything is physically okay.

Also, low estrogen (which can result from breastfeeding) can decrease your level of natural lubrication, making sex difficult or painful. This can be effectively treated by your doctor and/or ameliorated by lots of lube.

SCHEDULE TIME TOGETHER

I have been resistant to this idea forever, but my husband finally convinced me this past January that we should make a resolution to schedule the right conditions for sex. It doesn't mean we have to just do it because it's Friday, but it means we schedule the time to be together on Friday that leads to the relaxation and reconnection that makes it more likely that we (okay, *me*) will want to do it.

"The reason why scheduling time together works," says Savage, "is that there's no burden to perform. If sex happens, great. If not, hold each other, watch TV, talk. It's the pressure that kills sex, so schedule intimacy."

REMEMBER THIS IS A MOMENT IN TIME

You have your whole relationship ahead of you. "If things change in your sex life right now, it doesn't mean it's going away forever," says Martinez. "It just means that right now it's not going to be the same as it was before."

GET HELP IF YOU NEED IT

"I would encourage couples not to think of talking to a sex therapist as something being broken but approach it more like, 'How do we make this transition?'" says Martinez, who sees couples for a whole host of reasons, including painful sex, mismatched expectations, and—usually—a lack of communication. And that's what she (and others like her) are there for, to hear from both of you in a safe, neutral environment and help you find your way back to each other.

"I have two sofas in my office," says Martinez. "When people come in and sit on opposite sofas, it's usually because they should have come in a lot earlier." To find a therapist in your area, check out page 376.

Been There, Done That: Moms Talk About Sex in Early Parenthood

I was cleared at four weeks, but there's no way in hell I was having sex. I had lots of stitches.
—AMANDA, SAN DIEGO, CALIFORNIA

During the entire time that I was breastfeeding, I had zero sex drive. For each of my kids, that meant it was almost a year after childbirth before I was interested in sex in any way, shape, or form. We did what we could. If we had [vaginal] sex, lubrication was a must, but for the most part we got creative and figured out other things to do.
—MOM OF FOUR IN NORTH CAROLINA

It took me two months to even get my mirror out and look at my vagina. I was scared she had changed. Getting my vagina back was way more important than getting my body back. I wanted to possess her again as sexy, hot, and desirable. It was like having your new Mercedes get into a fender bender. You're like, "OMG, what happened to this amazing thing!"   —SND, ATLANTA, GEORGIA

No interest in sex. Husband was very frustrated. It was a constant, terrible struggle. He didn't understand that my

body didn't belong to me anymore: it had been an incubator, a dairy bar, forklift, plaything, blanket, and so on. The last thing I wanted was to use it to serve another human's needs.   —ANONYMOUS

We found since we couldn't have sex for the first six weeks that shared showers really helped keep us connected.

—KAITLYNN, MANITOBA, CANADA

My advice is to be patient and both try to have an understanding that the body needs to heal. After that, schedule regular sex so that neither of you feels neglected.

—MOM TO TWO IN HOUSTON, TEXAS

It took many months to feel 100 percent like my old self down there. Breastfeeding struggles and the demands of a newborn made me feel pretty "touched out." We talked a lot about it. Sometimes snuggling was enough for him. Sometimes that alone was a sacrifice for me. I found that when I refueled my tank, I had more energy for my husband. Explaining this to him really helped us. I needed "me time" first, and then I could make "us time." He was always willing to give me "me time" once he understood that!

—ANONYMOUS

How to Feel Good About Childcare

Figuring out who will care for your child while you are at work can be a huge source of stress, both from a logistical standpoint—researching daycares and getting on waitlists, finding recommended nannies and interviewing them thoroughly—and from an emotional standpoint: feeling comfortable with someone else caring for your baby.

The good news is that "a huge compendium of studies that looked at early childhood development found that there was no hugely significant difference between daycare and someone staying home with the baby," says Lauren Smith Brody, who did extensive research on childcare for her book *The Fifth Trimester: The Working Mom's Guide to Style, Sanity, and Big Success After Baby.*

What matters, says anthropologist Sarah Hrdy, PhD, is the kind of family support a child has and how responsive other caregivers are to your infant's needs. "Those were better predictors of developmental outcomes like self-control, respect for others, and social compliance than actual time spent away from the mother."

Whatever choice you make, when you have good people caring for your child, they can become a professional resource that helps you manage transitions and troubleshoot issues related to feeding, sleeping, and more. They will not only be part of your child's community, but they can be part of your parenting team.

HERE ARE A FEW WAYS TO FEEL GOOD ABOUT CHILDCARE

Spend Some Time with Caregiver(s) Before Committing

Once you have chosen a daycare center, ask if you can come back and observe on another day, recommends Brody. Watch how the caregivers interact with all the kids (including the older ones) so you can see what your child's future looks like there. You will see more of what the center is really like when you are there for an extended period of time and can be a fly on the wall.

Before signing a contract with a sitter, have her do a trial period with you for a few days. You can stay home at first to see her interact with your baby and show her your schedule, but eventually, you can do a trial run by heading out for some time to yourself.

Start Childcare a Week Early

Whatever arrangement you go with—your mother-in-law, a daycare center, or a sitter—start a week before you will be returning to work. That way you can do some short days to give everyone time to adjust to the new normal. You can also practice and fine-tune your getting-out-of-the-house routine, have some time to yourself to take care of things (maybe shop for a new work outfit or get a haircut?), and, when you see how he is adjusting, you will start that first day back without jitters about his situation.

What If I Feel Guilty?

You won't be alone. A lot of women say they feel guilty leaving their child to be cared for by someone other than themselves. And guilt is a common feeling among moms, usually tied to the pressures that we put on ourselves or that society puts on us (more about that in the last section of the book). Some of us may feel guilty about leaving our kids to go to a job outside the home, and others may not feel guilty about going back to work but then feel guilty about not feeling guilty!

"I always ask moms to get curious about the sources of the messages that fuel their guilt," says New York psychotherapist Sarah Best. "Very often, the messages are ideas that the moms themselves don't actually endorse. Getting clear about those ideas and then consciously rejecting them can be incredibly helpful."

Brody found that women for whom work is a financial imperative feel less guilt about putting their children in daycare than women who do not have similar financial constraints. If you are returning to work for reasons beyond a paycheck, give those reasons equal weight to your family's finances and see if that helps relieve your concern.

You Are Building Your Child's Community

Childcare serves a very practical purpose. It enables you to work to take care of your family financially and, in an ideal world, to take care of yourself personally. But when you can understand that it does something deeper than that, it will help you feel even better about it.

A woman I really trust once told me, "The more people who love your child, the better." And that woman was my mom. I have thought of that again and again since becoming a parent. When I leave my kids with other people, I find it reassuring to think about the fact that I am helping to build their community and growing the number of people who love and care for them and will look out for them when I am not there. Many of the daycare providers and sitters who have taken care of my children over the years have come to be like family, and transitioning out of their care was a bittersweet life passage.

Caregivers Can Give Your Children Things You Can't (Or Don't Want To)

We all have different strengths, and outside caregivers will have strengths different from yours and can share those with your child. For instance, I kinda suck at art, but both my children seem to have a natural interest and ability in it. We have somehow landed a stream of sitters who are amazing artists and have helped my children develop and follow those abilities.

Another area of parenting in which I have little interest is imaginary play, but it is the favorite way for both of my children to spend their time. One of our sitters will spend *hours* entering into all kinds of imaginary worlds—running stuffy "hospitals" and "schools," playing family, setting up a "train" to travel across the country in the "olden times." Knowing that they get these solid chunks of time to indulge and develop that part of their creativity gives me great peace of mind when I just can't muster the interest on the weekend. (Thank you, NA!)

What If I Miss My Child's Milestones?

"A lot of women worry about missing out on their babies' 'firsts,'" says Lori Mihalich-Levin, author of *Back to Work After Baby*. "But the reality is you could be attached to your baby all day, every day, and still miss a first. He could learn how to clap in his crib in the middle of the night, and the first time you see them reach a milestone, it will be a first for you."

If this is something that is really concerning you, Mihalich-Levin recommends asking your childcare provider to keep those moments to themselves and let you discover them on your own. "Your baby will develop at her own pace," and you can revel in it whenever it becomes something that happens in your presence. It will also be wonderful when you have a caregiver—at daycare or at home—who is just excited as you to see your child take big leaps in development."

Your Comfort Is What Matters

What the research shows, says Brody, is that what was more important than the type of care setting parents chose for their child (assuming it is a safe, well-run place or person) was the comfort level the parents had with it. The more comfortable you are, the more comfortable your kid will be and the happier your development as a family. "So," advises Brody, "make a decision that feels as emotionally right for you as it is logistically right."

Been There, Done That: Moms Share How They Made Decisions About Childcare

---

My husband and I are both very happy with center-based childcare, and found an abundance of acceptable options with warm, play-based environments and energetic teachers with CPR training. We learned so much from them. They've helped raise a lot more babies than I have. They're really the ones who taught us how to use bottles, how to engage with a child who can't sit up, how to respond in hard moments. I never saw them as competition or suspicious, outside influences. They were more people to love my child, and they came with a deep body of knowledge. I'm profoundly grateful to all of them.

—JAMIE, ATLANTA, GEORGIA

I chose a nanny because I had twins, so it cost about the same to hire a nanny as it did to send two littles to daycare. I like the idea of her being a "second mother" whom they are totally comfortable with. She is also able to take them after hours, when my husband and I have to travel, and once a week in the evenings to give us a date night.

—MEIMEI, HONOLULU, HAWAII

We went with an in-home daycare, where one woman (and a helper) took care of six to eight kids at her house. The woman pretty much became another member of our family.

We chose this type of care initially for the cost, but we also felt that it was good for babies. They still got to interact with other children but got more individual attention than they might have at a center.

—AMY, SHREWSBURY, MASSACHUSETTS

We chose for our daughter to go to daycare. We love the idea of her being around a lot of different children and learning from them. She loves where she is. I often have to pry her hands off the doorjamb just to get her to leave!

—JENNIFER, ATLANTA, GEORGIA

Your Game Plan for Returning to Work

You will likely have a lot of emotions about returning to work—some of them conflicting. You may feel sad to leave your baby. You may feel relief to let a professional (or professionals) be in charge of baby care while you return to a job you have some idea how to do. (And then you may feel guilt over that relief!) You might be anxious about leaving your child in the care of someone else (see "How to Feel Good About Childcare" on page 282). Maybe you're angry that your workplace doesn't offer more (or any) leave.

Whatever you are feeling makes total sense. This is a big transition, and the research shows that—for many women—the return to work happens before they are ready and is harder than they expect.

That's what Lauren Smith Brody discovered while researching her book *The Fifth Trimester*. The name comes from Brody's realization that "there was a whole other developmental stage that moms went through" when they returned to work. She took the idea from Harvey Karp, author of überpopular *The Happiest Baby on the Block*.

Karp calls the first twelve weeks of a baby's life the fourth trimester and advises parents to "'just get to twelve weeks and your baby will connect to you and it will be such a great feeling,'" says Brody. "But I knew that twelve weeks was when I would be going back to work (and that I had a much better maternity leave situation than most women), so the irony of that just kind of hit me."

But when Brody returned to work, she discovered that the difficulty of the adjustment "was just a season to get through," and the research she conducted with other working moms confirmed it. She surveyed nearly one thousand working moms in every kind of field and job, and what she found was that "on average, women said they were feeling physically better after birth by about 5.5 months and that they were feeling emotionally a little bit better by 5.8 months."

"What that said to me is that there is very, very definitively a fifth trimester—a developmental period in which these women were still preparing for (and also launching into) new motherhood," says Brody. "And almost no one was physically home with their baby at that moment. Women were returning to work before they were emotionally ready."

HOW TO MAKE THIS TRANSITION AS COMFORTABLE AS POSSIBLE

Hash Out the Logistics

Just getting to work is going to involve a whole new routine that may involve packing baby bags or leaving sets of directions, working in a last feed, possibly schlepping a breast pump or even a baby if your child will be attending daycare near your work. Lori Mihalich-Levin recommends brainstorming how the mornings and the evenings will work and coming up with a starter plan. Yes, you will learn things right away (and then over time) that will alter it, but it can make you feel more at ease to have a preliminary routine in place.

Bring Your Baby to Work Before You Start Back

Brody, who returned to her executive-level job as an editor at *Glamour* magazine after her first son was born, recommends bringing your baby to work—if it's even a remotely baby-friendly space—before you return. Doing so enables you to blend your worlds a little and makes your new reality visible to your coworkers. Plus, babies are made to attract people, so it's likely he will soon have a fan club around him and you'll build in some goodwill by introducing your son to even your most taciturn colleagues. Plus, you'll get to show him where you will be spending your time and explain why. Of course, he won't understand, but you will and that's what matters.

Do a Childcare Trial Run (but Then Get a Haircut)

Whatever morning routine you come up with, try it out one or more days before you actually have to be at work. This enables you to ease into your childcare situation (see "How to Feel Good About Childcare" on page 282), practice the routine to see what works and tweak it, and, then—*bonus!*—you can go have a few hours by yourself to get a haircut or whatever else will help you feel good about entering the world of no pajamas and daily showers.

Start Back Midweek

That first week back is going to be exhausting. Starting back on a Thursday, if you can swing it, will get you that much closer to a weekend where you can rest and think about what worked in those first two days logistically and what will help for your first full week.

Return Gradually If Possible

If you can use a little bit of your leave to have a few days off in the first weeks back, consider a part-time schedule that enables you to get used to being away from your baby and to your new routine. For instance, Brody suggests thinking about cutting your leave short by a week and then taking those five days and using them to be at home for the first five Fridays of your return.

Consider Working from Home If It Might Be an Option

After my first daughter was born, my work was willing to let me work from home one day a week, which not only made the transition easier but helped me keep my milk supply up, since I had three days of breastfeeding and four days of pumping.

"If you ask to work from home, come up with a plan of how it will work," advises Brody. "Show how you will meet your deliverables, make it clear that you will have childcare in place, and include a date to reassess the arrangement. It will help your boss feel more comfortable if he or she doesn't think it is forever." Of course, if it's going well . . .

FIND SUPPORT AMONG WORKING MOMS

"When I was pregnant and when I was on leave, I had great support through my local yoga studio, prenatal classes, and moms' groups," says Lori Mihalich-Levin, "but they were not necessarily working moms." When Mihalich-Levin went back to work, she found there were a lot of working moms in the office, none of whom were talking about their experiences and providing support to each other. So she created what she calls her "working moms' posse," inviting these women to lunch once a month and creating an online discussion forum for them to share their experiences, concerns, and advice. "It really changed the connectedness of the parents where I work," says Mihalich-Levin.

Check to see if your office already has something like this, and, if not, consider starting a group. Or, if that seems like too much right now, just invite one or more working moms out to lunch or take a coffee break with them in your first week back and ask them how they made the transition. You can build from there.

See page 377 for online working moms' groups you can join.

WORKING THROUGH "I HAVE TO QUIT"

"Every woman I surveyed—no matter her career or level of ambition—said that she had a moment of feeling like she 'had to quit,'" says Brody. "Some women felt that way for months. Others might have just had one really bad morning when it all came to a head."

For many moms, quitting is just not an option, and for those who can make a change, those early months of working-mom adjustment are not the best time to make that decision, says Brody. Most of the women felt the compulsion to quit when they were still in that developmental transition—what

Brody calls the fifth trimester—and hadn't yet made it to the other side to make a more settled and informed choice.

Looking at research on endurance, Brody found a few ways to work through those initial moments when you feel like leaving your job is the only solution (even if it's not an option):

- Realize the transition you are going through is finite.
- Make a list of what you get out of your job (and, yes, a paycheck counts).
- Make a list of what you bring to your workplace (this can help you feel more at peace with the personal compromises you feel you are making for your job, says Brody).
- Acknowledge your new learning curve. While you may be returning to a job you know how to do, you are now learning how to be a working mom. You are not going to hit a home run (or maybe even make contact with the ball) for a good, long while.
- Celebrate small successes. For Brody, this can mean writing something on your to-do list that you've already done, just so you can cross it off to feel a sense of accomplishment.
- Be patient. "Try not to make any major decisions for three months," says Brody.

SEE YOUR RETURN AS A CAREER OPPORTUNITY

Though it may not happen in the early weeks or even months of your return, once you are settled into your life as a working mom, "you will become infinitely more efficient," says Mihalich-Levin, who recommends that women look at their return to work "through a leadership lens, because you walk away from becoming a parent with so many newly developed skills that you can be using in the workplace."

Brody was surprised to discover that her return to work "was a time of real growth in my career and at home, and it was striking to feel that growth in a time when I had felt so desperate."

In our culture of inadequate support for working parents, it is easy to feel apologetic about taking leave or having to cut out in time for daycare pickup or missing a meeting to pump, but remember what you are bringing back to the job: a whole set of new skills, a developing ability to multitask like a master, and the incentive to work as efficiently as possible. You are valuable to your workplace and will only grow more so as you settle into this new phase of your life. Don't apologize for raising a person and doing a paid job. Brag about it. You are freaking awesome.

Been There, Done That: Moms Talk About the Return to Work After Baby

---

I stayed at home full-time for the first four months and nearly lost my mind. I was sobbing hysterically one day at about three months in when I realized that I had to get back to work. I felt I'd lost my identity. I was so happy when my nanny started working forty hours a week. I'm a much better mother as a working mother who gets a break from my kids.

—MEIMEI, HONOLULU, HAWAII

I wish I'd tried to set expectations with my boss ahead of time and that I'd requested a chance to reassess a few months later. What worked at three months wasn't necessarily the best setup at six months, nine months, or later.

—JAMIE, ATLANTA, GEORGIA

I took a full two months off and then the third month we switched off, so I worked Monday, Wednesday, and Friday and watched the kid Tuesday, Thursday while my partner worked. My son started daycare on the day he turned three months. Going back to work full-time was hard because I missed him, but I enjoyed being back in the swing of things.

—DONNA, DECATUR, GEORGIA

I always tell people on the fence about work versus being a SAHM [stay-at-home mom] that you may not know how you will feel until you've actually been back at work. Some people return to work and are surprised to realize they wish they hadn't, and some return to work and are surprised to realize how glad they are they are working.

—ANONYMOUS

PART III

Staying Strong

*The Big Picture of
Motherhood*

Who Am I Now?

That's a damn good question. Are you the person you used to be? Is that person gone forever? Are you some totally new person? Is *Mom* your entire identity now? Are you a hybrid? Do you feel comfortable in your new skin? Do you miss your old self? Do you feel like an impostor in this new role? Do you feel like this was what you were born to do? Does your identity as a mom fit you like a glove? Is that a good thing? Some gloves are kinda tight. Do you wonder why they use that analogy to talk about things fitting well? Do you wish I would stop asking questions and start the chapter?

IT'S OKAY TO STRUGGLE

"Some people very easily and quickly make the jump into motherhood and their identity as a mother," says Carla Naumburg, PhD, author of *Parenting in the Present Moment: How to Stay Focused on What Really Matters.* "And for other people it really is a struggle. And if it's a struggle for you, that's okay. Don't make it harder by beating yourself up for it. It doesn't mean that you are a bad mother or that you're screwing this up. It's just part of going through a big change in life."

Amen, sister.

For me, the transition to motherhood—postpartum anxiety aside—felt fairly natural. I had always wanted to be a mom, and I felt good being one pretty much right away. The piece that has been hard for me? Accepting the different body I have after two pregnancies and two deliveries.

On the one hand, motherhood has given me the opportunity to put worrying about how I look at the bottom of the priority pile, which has been liberating. But on the other, I struggle with feeling disconnected from something that used to be a big part of my identity—feeling really good about how I looked. I'm not saying this is a lofty part of me, but it is part of me, and it's where I struggle when it comes to my identity in motherhood. I have struggled to accept the new body I live in, and getting comfortable with it means saying goodbye to something that used to be really important to me.

"A good friend once said to me, up until you had a baby, you spent your whole life weaving a beautiful rug with lots of colors representing who you are and patterns that represent your experience," says Nitzia Logothetis, founder and chairwoman of the Seleni Institute (where I work as editorial director). "And then you have a baby and the rug disintegrates and you have to start weaving it again." Got your shuttle ready? (That's a weaving reference, FYI.)

GRIEF CAN BE A NATURAL PART OF THE PROCESS

"When women are pregnant, no one talks to them about how the life they are living is no longer going to be what it was," says Jerilyn Brownstein, MSW, who facilitates workshops, retreats, and support groups for mothers in New Paltz, New York, and New York City. "There's no goodbye ceremony during pregnancy. There's 'the baby is coming' ceremony, but there is no ritual to say goodbye to the life you had as a woman and as a couple." And without that preparation, says Brownstein, a lot of women can feel blindsided by the disorientation they may feel in their new role. "When a woman becomes a mother, there is a birth," says Brownstein. "But there is also a death, and that death goes unrecognized and underground."

"Grief is a huge part of the process of becoming a mom," agrees Kate Lynch Bieger, PhD, a psychologist in New York City who specializes in perinatal mental health and parenting and who attended one of Brownstein's motherhood groups. "Women who become mothers may be grieving their old life; moms going back to work may be grieving being at home with their baby. You gain something, but there's loss every step of the way. I can't tell you how often I have moms come in those first few months of motherhood feeling such a loss of their life before. Not knowing where they are and what happened to them. It's reassuring for them to know that it's normal to be out there in rough waters, in new territory."

NAVIGATING THE NEW TERRITORY
OF MOTHERHOOD

You *are* in new territory. You are experiencing things you never have before (even if you already have a child, because every child is different and a family changes as it grows). Some of them can be so beautiful and unparalleled, like feeling the fuzz of a one-month-old's head right under your chin as you cuddle in bed or hearing your baby laugh for the first time, being called "Mama," being one of the most important people on the planet to another human. (What a power trip!)

But there are other experiences that are less beautiful. Like discovering how incredibly irritable you become when you are sleep deprived. Or looking across the couch at your partner and realizing you haven't really looked in his or her eyes for days, maybe weeks. Or feeling like your body has become an unknown thing to you.

Any number of the challenges we've covered in this book are part of this shift, and it is the terrain on which you are charting a new course for yourself and your family.

"Eventually, you will settle," says Naumburg, "but you want the interim to not feel painful. So, the question is, how do you want to get support through it?"

PUT YOURSELF FIRST

That's weird advice for a new mom, but "it's absolutely necessary," says Hara Ntalla, MS Ed, the clinical director of the Seleni Institute. "When you recharge, your baby will recharge. When you make your well-being a priority, you show your child that this is important and necessary for everyone to do."

What does that mean practically? Do things with your young child that you enjoy doing. Bring her along for your favorite activities, and take breaks from her and reconnect with friends and activities from your pre-baby life.

JOIN A MOMS' SUPPORT GROUP

Finding a moms' group that is either facilitated by a professional such as Brownstein or is casually organized gives you a place to share what you are going through and hear that you are not alone. There is real power in having your experiences validated and seeing that your adjustment to motherhood—whatever it looks like—is normal. A good moms' group where you feel comfortable (and, if you don't, look for another) can be a safe space to share all your feelings without worrying about someone thinking you're crazy or that you don't like being a mom. See page 258 for how to find a moms' group that will be a helpful and safe space for you.

BE HONEST

If you have not picked up on it by now, I'm pretty open about my struggles as a mom. I've been that way from the first party I went to after my first daughter was born. It was a holiday party with my husband's coworkers from *The New York Times*. One of the younger ones—newly married and in her twenties—came up to me and asked giddily, "How is motherhood?"

"Hard," I answered. "Really, really hard." She wasn't expecting *that* answer! But you know what? She said it was refreshing to hear someone be honest. But there have been times when my candor has found no solidarity.

I remember an essay I wrote and shared with my friends called "The Bittersweet Loneliness of New Motherhood." The piece talked about how I feel ultimately responsible for my children's well-being and how it was a privilege and a burden at the same time and that felt lonely. The friends I emailed it to did not "get it." One even told me how her husband is such an active co-parent that she could not relate at all (ouch!).

But you know what? When I finally published that piece on *The Huffington Post*, comment after comment (most of them along the lines of "Yes! This!" or "I thought it was just me" or "Oh my god, this is so true") demonstrated that I was not alone. My first sample size had just been too small.

"I think a part of our culture that is diseased is that there is no safe and sacred space to share your taboo material," says Brownstein (like, say, the fact that you are not enjoying motherhood the way everyone thinks you should). Guess what? This book is an effort to change that culture, and you can join the crusade!

GET DEEP

As I said, Brownstein looks at motherhood as an initiation experience (kind of like birth). "I can't think of another experience in the natural world that meets it other than death," says Brownstein. "So it's a big one."

That sounds kind of dramatic—maybe even scary—but Brownstein's whole point is that if, as a society, we could acknowledge that loss and change and struggle and happiness are all part of this big transition, we could be more accepting of all of it. And then it becomes way *less* scary.

APPROACH IT AS A PROCESS

"It can take years to build up what it is to be a mother," says Bieger. And that applies to all parts of this new life, from your body to your relationships, and beyond.

I interviewed Jane Marie, a writer and radio producer who works on *This American Life*, among other shows, about the changing relationship you have to your body when you become a mom, and she put it in a pretty beautiful way. "You're going to spend a couple of years at least going through a transformation," she told me. "My daughter is three and she likes bugs, so we talk a lot about caterpillars turning into butterflies. We talk a lot about my body being a chrysalis and about how she has changed, but I'm changing too."

"As a society, we've become so impatient. When we struggle with something, we expect to have the answers immediately," says Logothetis. "But identity is something that is continuously evolving. Don't be frightened by feelings of ambivalence. Know that it's a process and that you'll come to a conclusion, but it might take time."

APPRECIATE IT AS AN EDUCATION

"It's a really rich time to learn about yourself and your kids," says Logothetis. "To learn about your abilities and your emotional trigger points, what you enjoy, what you don't enjoy, and what you can learn to enjoy. And your children's identities are shifting too, so there's always a learning curve."

LET YOUR GOAL BE ACCEPTANCE

"We have to continually reaccept parts of ourselves when we go through different experiences," says Christina Hibbert, PsyD, a clinical psychologist in Flagstaff, Arizona, who specializes in women's mental health and motherhood. "Every phase of your life you have new doubts and new questions about yourself. A lot of people misunderstand acceptance and think it means we have to like or agree with something. Acceptance can just be 'This is how I am right now. I can change it if I want, but I am not going to fight myself over it.'"

REPLACE SELF-ESTEEM WITH SELF-WORTH

"Identity and self-worth underlie every issue that mothers come to talk to me about," says Hibbert. In our society, so often the focus is on building a person's self-esteem, but Hibbert shifts the focus to self-worth. "Self-esteem is about how we think about ourselves, what we do, how 'good' we are at things, and how people perceive us. All of those things shift, and we don't have a lot of control over them." So Hibbert talks to women about the value of self-worth, which involves knowing who you really are outside of what you think and do. "That can't be taken away by anybody."

CONSIDER PSYCHOTHERAPY

A relationship with a good therapist is a wonderful tool for weathering all the storms—big and little—of life, and the normal adjustment to your role as a mom is one of them. "You get to go into a room for a period of time and there is a person who just wants to listen to you, is highly skilled in listening to you, and then you can walk out and leave it there," says Naumburg. "You have a place where you can deal with it, but you don't have to think about it all the time."

That can be invaluable for a mom who is otherwise

spending most of her waking hours worrying about taking care of other people. "Therapy can be a form of self-care," says psychotherapist Ariel Flavin. "You deserve to give yourself every tool and support that you can benefit from and even enjoy." See page 373 for tips on finding a good one for you.

LOOK FORWARD

No matter how many headlines tell you how to "get your body back," there is no going "back." There is only now and what is to come. "Instead of thinking, 'I have to get back to who I was,'" says Brownstein. "You have to go forward into who you're becoming."

So let's do it.

Been There, Done That: Moms Talk About Their Identity Now

Having kids has made me feel more connected to the world—like I have a bigger stake in the universe.

—Nicole, Brooklyn, New York

I feel like I lost myself a bit when I became a mom. It was as if what was "me" had just left the building! What helped was starting to fight for the things that give me joy, not because anyone doesn't want me to have them but because there are so many other demands on my time and attention.

—Emily, New York

I think I became more of me with motherhood. I'm more aware, more loving, more organized, but I'm also more worried, more exhausted, and more cautious.

—JEN, PORTLAND, OREGON

Suddenly, I was in mothers' clubs, and I actually took comfort in identifying as a mom. Sometimes I worry that I rely too much on this—when I'm someplace without kids, I can feel a bit lost.   —KRISTEN, SAN FRANCISCO, CALIFORNIA

Being a mom has changed my relationship to gender norms. I'm a lesbian and have never been particularly feminine-looking or gender-conforming. Before I was a mom, I was pretty content to be on the periphery of female experience. Being a mom has brought me squarely into female experience in a way that is both exciting (I can now talk to and relate to a much wider set of women than before; I feel part of a club I always felt pretty excluded from before), and alienating (I now compare myself to other women/moms in a way that actually makes me feel even more marginalized because I don't conform to stereotypical gender norms).

—JULIE, SAN FRANCISCO, CALIFORNIA

I'm a confident person who is way more concerned about social justice and making the world a better place. I didn't know why I was living before kids. Being a mom has been the most wonderful, natural thing to ever happen to me.

—JENNIFER, ATLANTA, GEORGIA

While I have always been and always will be "me," the responsibilities associated with being the best me I can be for

these people I have created brings out sides of me that were dormant. It brings out the best in me and simultaneously the least patient. —KAREN, ROCKVILLE, MARYLAND

My identity changed and continues to change the longer I parent. The initial transition was a shock—physically, mentally, and emotionally. The exhaustion of labor and childbirth, coupled with the totally draining process of caring for an infant, wiped me out. The first year, in fact, was a blur. As my kids have become more independent, I've found it keeps getting better.

—MARGARET, BROOKLYN, NEW YORK

The Most Important Person

Once upon a time, there was a writer and mom named Kate Rope who wanted to write a book about how moms can prioritize their emotional health and truly take care of themselves. She had recovered from one very difficult pregnancy and two bouts of postpartum anxiety. She'd weaned off her antidepressant medication and learned how to manage her anxiety. She wanted to share with other women the things she'd learned and the people she had met on that journey. So she took her editor out to lunch and sold her on a book idea!

Then one day—soon after that—Kate's husband got a great job in a new city, and they moved their entire family to a new state. Kate was excited for the move, but—three months into it—she was paralyzed by anxiety again. She found her way to the offices of a psychiatrist who recommended she go back on antidepressant medication to weather the transition (turns out these are very hard for Kate, as they are for many of us). She also found a fitness boot camp with an incredible community—a workout experience so fulfilling and enjoyable she happily woke up every morning at 5:30 to do it. She realized that she had the tools to prioritize her physical and emotional health, and this was the time to do it.

So Kate got on the horn to her editor and told her what had been happening—that between the adjustment to her new life, her part-time job, and the fact that she was regularly exercising for the first time since becoming a mom, she just didn't see how she was going to make her book deadline. That it would be hypocritical to write a book telling moms why they should prioritize taking care of themselves if she didn't practice what she preached. That she had to move her deadline back *by a year.*

You know what? That awesome editor said she completely understood. And they are both living normally ever after.

The moral of the story? Put yourself first.

But don't just take it from me.

"The most important relationship you will ever have in your life is the relationship you have with yourself," says Graeme Seabrook, an internationally certified life coach in Charleston, South Carolina, who experienced anxiety and PTSD after her first son was born. "Your kids will move away eventually—and we all hope that the partners we have will be with us our whole lives, but crazy stuff happens! The only person who is going to be with you until you die and who has been with you since you were born is you."

We are the only part of our lives that we have total control over and total responsibility for. "But, as women, we drop that responsibility," says Seabrook. "We kick it away. We *run* from it in the name of serving other people."

That isn't good for us, but it also isn't good for anyone else.

"It doesn't work," says Seabrook. "It does not make your relationship stronger, it does not make your children happier, and it does not make your friendships better.

"On the flip side," continues Seabrook, "when you put yourself in the center of your life and think 'How can I be healthier and happier?' everything else starts to fall into place, because moms are generally the lynchpin of the family. The better we work, the better everything else works."

IF YOU WON'T DO IT FOR YOU, DO IT FOR YOUR KID(S)!

"The thing that is clearest to me now—having kids who are seventeen and twenty—is that the one and only thing that actually matters and makes a difference when it comes to being a parent is being in the best place you can be as a person," says Judith Warner, author of *Perfect Madness: Motherhood in the Age of Anxiety.* Warner has interviewed hundreds of mothers over the past fifteen years of being a journalist and says with certainty that the best thing you can do as a parent is to "identify the toxic stresses in your life and address them. Take care of yourself physically and mentally."

That's the argument Kate Lynch Bieger, PhD, makes when she works with moms in her psychotherapy practice in New York City. "It can be so hard for moms to prioritize themselves," says Bieger, "and so I say this so many times a week to people sitting on my couch: 'If you are not taking care of yourself, you are not going to be fully there for anyone else.'"

PAY ATTENTION TO RED FLAGS

I hope by now you are convinced that real self-care should be a regular practice, but let's say you're not. Or let's say you're human and even though you try to practice it, you fall behind because life got crazy. (Who, me? Never!) If—or when—either of those things is true, be on the lookout for the red flags that remind you to return to taking care of yourself.

"For some, it's snapping at her kids or yelling too much," says Bieger. For me, it's usually a feeling of overwhelming exhaustion. Spending time with my kids starts to feel like a chore. I begin resenting my husband. Martyr syndrome creeps in.

"When you experience a digging in of the heels, a feeling of 'I just can't take care of myself,' that's when you need it most," says Bieger.

FIGURE OUT WHAT YOU NEED TO FEEL WHOLE

Think back over your whole life—childhood, high school, college, dating, this pregnancy you just finished. What were the things you did that made you feel good? What is the thing you have always done that brings you back to yourself in times of stress?

Is there a hobby you have been neglecting? Have you noticed that the times you felt the most stable in your life were when you had an exercise routine? Do you miss reading fiction? Does your church, temple, or meditation center ground you? Is your bathtub a place you like to escape to? Does a cup of coffee and a deep chat with a close friend restore you? Is being in nature like pressing a reset button? Remember when you did yoga? Didn't it make you feel great? Do you miss glee club?

You get the idea.

If you have not had something that was all yours, something that relieved stress, "refilled your bucket" (as my daughter's preschool teacher would put it), made you feel whole and at peace, now is a great time to find out what does. What sounds good to you? This is another area (like exercise) where trial and error is your friend.

Of course, when we're talking about early parenthood, you will likely need to start small and then build up. You don't need one more thing on your to-do list that you are not getting to (if you're in the immediate postpartum period, you don't even need a to-do list).

Right now, my weekly fiddle lessons are my favorite time of the week, but my kids are ages ten and six, and I sleep through the night. When they were babies, it was a weekly spin class if I could get there. Of course, we know by now that this book is aimed to help you avoid the pitfalls of my early pregnancies and postpartum periods, so I'd aim for something more regular (even if it has to be for a shorter period of time).

A Small List of Big Ways to Take Care of Yourself
- A regular religious or spiritual practice
- Yoga
- Exercise (see page 240)
- Hiking
- Reading
- Adult coloring books
- Arts and crafts

- Zoning out to your favorite TV show (yes, experts told me this qualifies)
- Playing or learning a musical instrument
- Joining a singing group
- Knitting or crocheting
- Improv classes
- Playing on a sports team
- Spending time in nature
- Going out dancing
- Dancing in your living room
- Napping
- Listening to music

It took until my kids were four and eight for me to realize that daily exercise has a life-changing effect on my energy and mood and ability to cope with life's stresses. Now I have become one of those people who used to annoy me—you know, those people who complain that they don't feel like themselves if they don't get a workout in? If you are one of those people, now I get you. If you are not, I get you too! The point is, it's never too late to learn how to make yourself feel good, and it is your job, when you have the energy, to do it. Unlike other elements of parenthood, you are the only one you can trust with it.

Been There, Done That: Moms Talk About Taking Care of Themselves

---

Finally going to yoga! Completely makes me feel like I have my life back, if only for that hour.

—BRANDY, CHICAGO, ILLINOIS

Karaoke and massage. They make everything better.

                    —JEN, PORTLAND, OREGON

I like to craft (when I have time!), read, and run.

                    —AMY, HOUSTON, TEXAS

By my second baby, I realized that I needed time to be able to go off by myself—to hike in the woods, sit in a coffee shop, read a book alone in bed all day. I took days off work when my kids were in daycare to have that time to myself.

                    —ANONYMOUS

The biggest change I've made to care for myself as a person is returning to the dance world. It has nothing to do with being a mother, and that's what makes it self-caring. It's reclaiming a part of my identity that had been set aside for a long time, and it's a tangible way for my kids to see me as more than just their mom. I feel more like a whole person, more like myself now.

                    —JESSICA, ATLANTA, GEORGIA

Beware the Cult of Perfect Motherhood

Our culture has a very complicated (and often hypocritical) relationship to motherhood. On the one hand, we place mothers on pedestals and tell them they have the most important job in the world. On the other hand, our society provides almost no institutional support for the endeavor of raising a child. From whom much is expected so little is given.

Our extended families are often far from us. There is no universal public or subsidized childcare. There is no national visiting nurse service for new moms. Parental leave is insufficient at best, nonexistent at worst. I am not trying to depress the hell out of you. Just trying to call a spade a spade. There is almost no institutional support for a job that is considered one of the most important you can undertake and that is certifiably one of the hardest you will ever have.

And yet, we place expectations that cannot possibly be met, even with incredible support. Expectations that don't even need to be met, because our children do better when they learn to rely on themselves and other members of their community. But that won't stop the culture at large from sending you one consistent, loud—but completely erroneous—message: it's all on you, and you gotta get it right.

OUR EPIDEMIC OF EXPECTATIONS

"We have this ideology of total motherhood," says Joan Wolf, PhD, associate professor women's and gender studies at Texas A&M University and author of *Is Breast Best?: Taking On the Breastfeeding Experts and the New High Stakes of Parenthood*, "which essentially tells women they are 100 percent responsible for the products they produce. We don't hold anybody on the planet accountable in that way for anything. We certainly don't hold fathers responsible in that way, and we don't hold governments or communities responsible."

"We are living in an epidemic of expectations," agrees Lauren Smith Brody, author of *The Fifth Trimester: The Working Mom's Guide to Style, Sanity, and Big Success After Baby*. "Women's expectations of themselves as workers and as mothers are just totally over the top. And, for me at least, it's the thing that pushes me over the edge. I find myself looking in the mirror and feeling like I am failing at everything."

The media and social media are filled with unrealistic images of celebrity (and real-life) moms doing it all and looking good doing it. "Our culture sets up these expectations that we are supposed to look amazing, be joyful, blissful, and happy, have amazing careers, and be perfect moms who have time for book club," says psychologist Kate Bieger. "That's an impossible expectation. You have to let go of your expectations and let it be what it really is."

. . . .

A Short History of the Conflicting and Overwhelming Expectations Placed on Mothers Through the Ages

. . . .

In her book *Perfect Madness: Motherhood in the Age of Anxiety*, journalist Judith Warner takes readers on a tour of advice given to—and expectations placed on—mothers over the past three hundred years. Turns out, from the time of the colonies—when mothers were held responsible for nothing less than their children's spiritual salvation—to the present day, mothers have been burdened with completely unrealistic and totally conflicting responsibilities. Let's take a quick trip through them.

- Keep yourself separate from your children
- Don't "coddle," "spoil," or "smother" your children
- Don't be "dangerously self-sacrificing"
- Avoid being anxious, overly concerned, or neurotic
- Make sure you are not "overattached"
- Create a "secure attachment" to your child
- Make sure you are not attached for the wrong reasons (for your needs, rather than your child's)
- Avoid "overbearing involvement"
- Be involved in your kids' lives!
- Enjoy your children!
- Meet your husband's needs—for your children's sake
- Break away from the identity of being a mother
- Be fulfilled—for yourself
- Be fulfilled—so you don't damage your kids' psyche
- Eschew motherhood all together

- Be happy so your children will be happy
- Don't work
- Work
- Have it all
- Build up your children's self-esteem
- Don't praise your children too much
- Stimulate early childhood learning starting in the womb
- Be "everything" to your children

Anybody else confused and exhausted?

YOU ARE NOT THE SUM OF YOUR CHOICES AND EXPERIENCES

The things you do or do *not* do in pregnancy (even *before* pregnancy), delivery, and early parenthood—breastfeeding, formula-feeding, having medication during delivery, using cloth diapers, attachment parenting, co-sleeping, crying it out, feeding your kid organic foods, letting your kid watch *Daniel Tiger*, working full-time, staying home full-time, and so on—are often seen as an indication of who you are as a person and mother instead of just choices you made or experiences you had along the way.

"These choices are labeled with this moral freight," says Wolf. "They indicate whether you are a person who cares about your child, whether you care about your health, whether you care about the environment. Pregnancy and motherhood have become this experience where any of your needs become irrelevant, and any potential risk you can eliminate for your child is worth it."

I mean, I've said that motherhood is a power trip, but that's a *lot* of power—way more than I think anyone would want and certainly way more than we actually have. But the messaging can make you second-guess or feel guilty about every choice you made or didn't make.

"Mothers have always been told that they are uniquely responsible for their children's well-being in the largest possible sense," says journalist Judith Warner. And that responsibility, says Warner, has roots in the individualism that defines America. So rather than looking to collective responsibility or social action to bear a large part of the responsibility of raising the next generation, we put it *all* on moms.

"We have a very individualized sense of what it means to succeed, and we have brought that orientation to motherhood," says Warner, who came of age in the 1980s in a generation "that was bathed in the ethos, 'You can do it! You can do it all! And you can do it single-handedly!'" And when those kinds of messages got filtered through the popular culture and media, says Warner, we ended up with "this emphasis on the mom and the extreme lengths women need to go to ensure their babies' health and well-being."

My radical hope for this book is that it can play a small role in giving a new generation of mothers the tools, permission, and road map for redefining what we expect of ourselves, how we take care of ourselves and our kids, and how we expect others—including government and institutions—to take care of us. To realize that what is being asked of us is not only unrealistic, but it is actually not *good* for us *or* our kids. I want us to start asking for better—from ourselves, our friends and family, and from our community.

Been There, Done That: Moms Talk About the Pressure to Be Perfect

There is so much out there about how to do it "right." I've always expected myself to "know better" and continue to punish myself for mistakes. Meanwhile, everyone around me tells me I'm a "great mom," but I feel like an impostor.
                                    —Jessica, Atlanta, Georgia

I know that "perfect" doesn't exist. It's an illusion. Parenting standards—what you must and should do—change every year anyway! I believe that the vast majority of us are doing the best we can, and most of our kids are going to turn out okay. Even if they don't, that probably doesn't have much to do with our parenting, which is just a small piece of the puzzle of who our kids turn out to be.
                                    —MeiMei, Honolulu, Hawaii

I have zero expectations on being perfect as a mom. I want my daughter to see me make mistakes so that she won't feel the pressure to be perfect herself, and so she can see ways to handle mistakes.   —Jennifer, Atlanta, Georgia

I was a young mom, and I felt that I needed to validate me being a good mom because some people around me judged my unplanned pregnancy as a mistake. However, after having huge issues with my husband, I completely re-evaluated my choices and decided to start doing things more because I liked and enjoyed them and because I be-

lieved they were the right choices for my family, rather than social pressure.   —PATTY, DECATUR, GEORGIA

Being a queer mom puts all your choices out there for public scrutiny. I am proud of my nontraditional family, but sometimes all the extra decisions and questions can be exhausting.   —MOLLY, MINNESOTA

Children have survived and become productive adults for centuries without an ounce of the ridiculous micromanagerial misery we currently tend to place on ourselves and them. And, really, the parents subscribing to the over-worry paradigm aren't the ones I'm concerned about. For the people who are likely to read this book: "Ladies, the kids are all right—mine and yours."

—KENDRA, ATLANTA, GEORGIA

Learning on the Job

I once called up one of my best mom friends to tell her about my latest "major parenting screwup." My daughter had been acting out, and I told my friend that "it's one of those times where it's taken me two weeks to realize how I need to handle the situation, and I've been doing it wrong until now." She paused and then answered matter-of-factly: "Isn't that just parenting?"

Yes, yes, it is. And that's why I love my friend Ariel, whose expertise as a therapist I have shared in other sections of this book.

Let's say you just got hired for a new job. It's a big promotion from your last position, and it comes with management responsibilities—which you've never had before—and requires skills that are almost all new to you. You were hired because of your passion and promise, not your track record. I'm guessing you would show up on the first day pretty nervous and aware that there were a lot of things you didn't know how to do. That you were going to learn on the job. That you were probably going to make a lot of mistakes and just hope none of them were too big.

That job is parenting, and yet somehow, making mistakes is not allowed. Particularly when it comes to moms. We are supposed to know what to do—to have a natural instinct for the job. I don't think it's an exaggeration to say that many of us expect near perfection straight out of the gate.

Moms sit on the couch across from psychologist Kate Bieger all the time and tell her that they have no idea what they are doing, but they are pretty sure the other moms do. "I let them in on the secret that I talk to a lot of moms and *none* of them do," says Bieger. "Everyone is learning on the job."

YOU ARE NEW TO ALL OF THIS

"So much of what I have learned has just been baptism by fire," says Jill Krause, mom to four and the creator of the honest and irreverent blog *Baby Rabies*. "You just get thrown into all these new situations." And you have to figure your way out of them by trial and error. That is the natural state of parenting. "I totally thought we were going to have it all together before we had kids," says Krause, "but when you think that way, the further you have to fall, so the sooner you can let yourself fall from grace, the better; it will be a shorter fall, and you will be all the better for it."

EMBRACE THE JOURNEY

If you have ever tried to "get something done" with a toddler, you have quickly discovered the frustration of spending the bulk of your time in the process and very little (none?) enjoying your accomplishment.

Kids love process. It's how they learn. Since she was little,

my older daughter has spent 75 percent of her playtime setting up the dollhouse, turning a room into the "olden times,"
building the LEGO town, deciding on everyone's made-up
cat names, and maybe 10 percent actually playing the game.
(I know that doesn't equal 100 percent, but there's a lot of
time unaccounted for in the life of a child.)

This is where children are like little Zen masters, showing
you—sometimes forcing you—to be present and realize that
the journey is where you will spend most of your time. If you
can see motherhood as a journey, rather than focusing on the
destination, you will find yourself far less frustrated and disappointed by the inevitable detours, flat tires, fender benders,
and times when you get completely lost.

"This is not a test where you get it right or you get it
wrong," says Bieger. "It's a process, and you get as much time
as you need to 'get it right.'"

CHANGE IS THE ONLY CONSTANT

Dana Rosenbloom, MS Ed, a wonderful parenting coach in
New York City, describes parenthood as a dance. "You are
going to make missteps, because you are talking about two
separate people who are growing and changing all the time,"
says Rosenbloom. "You will get into a rhythm that works for
a while and then it may not." Like the opening story in this
section, I've found that most phases of parenting—the really
smooth ones and the really bumpy ones—tend to last two weeks
before changing. And you can always count on that except
when you can't.

FOLLOW YOUR KID'S LEAD AND "LET IT GO!"

"As parents, when something goes wrong, we hold on to it and beat ourselves up over it," says Rosenbloom. "Take a lesson from your children. The next minute, they are on to something different. So, if you can, say, 'Okay, I totally screwed up that one, and it's a chance to step back, reassess, and move forward.' To beat yourself up over it is truly a waste of time, because your children have already moved on."

GIVE YOURSELF ROOM TO CHANGE

"When I became a mom, I was going to be the one who cloth diapers and breastfeeds and never lets them cry it out. There was a push to be a certain kind of mom," says Krause. "You were either A or B. But as things became more natural for me, I realized I'm kind of a hybrid. Give yourself permission to change. I'm a different mom with baby number four than I was for baby number one."

"There's this whole concept that it has to be set in stone," says Rosenbloom. "It doesn't. You can modify it. There's plenty of room for making it work for you in the moment where you are right now."

YOUR CHILD BENEFITS FROM YOUR EFFORT ALONE

Once again, parenting is a process, and the effort you put into it and the attention you show your child are all part of it even when that effort doesn't achieve your intended outcome. "Let's say your baby is having a digestive issue and you try one doctor, then a diet, then another—that's the work of parenting," says Rosenbloom. "And your child benefits just from the focus and love of someone trying to figure it out. The way your children understand your attachment to them is your responsiveness over the years. It's a combination of so many moments." But it is *not* any *one* moment.

MISTAKES ARE MOMENTS TO MODEL

No one moment is defining. No one moment is a point of no return. In fact, any moment of doing something as a parent that doesn't work out can be a moment when you model for your children what it is to be human, to not define learning experiences as "failure," to bounce back, to apologize and move forward, and that is a gift. "It is useful for children to see the full range of what humans experience," says Bieger. "We get to model that from now until forever."

"This is a profound lesson in accepting others, developing pro-social behavior, and being part of a trusting/trusted community," says Sarah Best, LCSW, a psychotherapist in New York City who specializes in reproductive mental health. "It's also what sets kids up to accept their own faults, which is essential for combating the perfectionism of the next generation!" Yes!

GO FOR A GROWTH MIND-SET

About ten years ago, a hot new idea hit the self-help bookshelf: the idea of "mind-set." Carol Dweck, PhD, now a professor of psychology at Stanford University, published the book *Mindset: The New Psychology of Success*, featuring research that showed that what matters when it comes to "success" is not as much natural skills or talents but the mind-set people bring to whatever skills or talents they have.

Those who have a "fixed" mind-set believe that abilities, skills, talents, intelligence, and the like are fixed traits that determine success and cannot be changed. Those who have a "growth" mind-set, on the other hand, believe that you can improve your abilities through work and dedication.

"A growth mind-set says you get better by effort and that mistakes are learning opportunities," says Debra Levy, MS Ed, PCC, a business and life coach in Arlington, Massachusetts. "The researchers found that people with a growth mind-set perform better, because they are more willing to take risks and learn."

Focus on the effort you are putting in, the risks you are taking, your willingness to learn and change and improve. Not "I'm a bad mom" or a "terrible mother" or even "a great mom." You are just a mom, and a person trying things out, taking risks, and continuously learning. "The growth mind-set says, 'I have more to learn,'" says Levy.

THERE ARE NO #PARENTINGFAILS

"The idea of 'failure' comes from a fixed mind-set," says Levy. "You either succeed or fail." When Levy works with her clients, she focuses on the lessons that can be learned when things *don't* go as you anticipated or wanted them to.

"It's trial and error, and, of course, we all have permission to be human," says Levy. And you deserve to be loved (by yourself and others) for the beautiful, imperfect human that you are. How boring would life be if everyone were perfect?

I think perhaps Rosenbloom put it best when she told

me during our interview, "It takes a whole lot to fuck up your kid."

Been There, Done That: Moms Talk About Learning on the Job

I used to think I had to get it right immediately. Now, I know it's a learning curve. I also used to think that one mistake obliterated all the good stuff, that if I ever fell off the perfect-parent wagon, I'd never be able to get back on again. But now I know that it's more about patterns than instances. If I am generally getting it right, I won't be penalized for periodic mistakes. My kid is tough, and so am I.

—Julie, San Francisco, California

I have honestly tried to fess up to my parenting errors when they occur by acknowledging them (to myself and to the kids) and apologizing. That way, I can also model that nobody is perfect and that there's a learning that comes from mistakes.

—Dagmar, Atlanta, Georgia

Unrealistic as it is, I expect no learning curve. In my professional life, I was much better at forgiving myself, learning, and moving on, but with mothering, I feel like there's too much at stake.   —Jessica, Atlanta, Georgia

I don't expect to get it right the first time. I make mistakes. A lot. I apologize. I show my kids that I make mistakes, that we all do. Making mistakes is not a bad thing. Not trying is far worse.   —Karen, Rockville, Maryland

A friend said to me, "Everything is a phase. A phase lasts no more than three weeks. You can handle anything for three weeks." While not entirely true, it's very helpful to have this frame of reference.

—Karen, Boston, Massachusetts

I raise my voice or check out for a bit sometimes. Is that a mistake? I think it is just being human. I want my kids to know and love me, *not some robot perfect mom.*

—Amanda, Portland, Oregon

Be Your Best Friend

You are putting so much effort into being good and kind to another being, and you are probably doing it without thinking too much about it. It may feel like second nature to care for this new person in the world who is trying to figure things out, but you know who else is trying to figure things out and find where she fits in? You. And you know who else deserves buckets of kindness and support and care while she does it? Yep, you guessed it. You.

"Make a goal to do one kindness for yourself each day," advises Christina Hibbert, PsyD, a clinical psychologist in Flagstaff, Arizona, who specializes in women's mental health and motherhood. "It doesn't have to be a big deal—it might be enjoying a piece of chocolate and putting on a TV show in your room for twenty minutes—but it's up to us to get it. Nobody is going to do it for you."

If you can't figure out what it is you need in a given moment, Hibbert recommends thinking about what you would do for someone else if you saw them struggling. "Thinking about what you would do for a friend is a perfect way to know what you want and need."

TALK TO YOURSELF AS CONSCIENTIOUSLY
AS YOU TALK TO YOUR KIDS

Chances are you give a lot of thought to the way you talk to your children when they spill a glass of milk, act out, are sad, when you are mad at them. If you're like me, there are many times when you don't manage to be as calm and kind in those moments as you want to be, but you think a lot about how to do better next time. It's an important area of assessment and improvement for you.

What about the way you talk to yourself? When my youngest daughter was three, she started calling herself "stupid" after she made mistakes. It was my husband who gently brought to my attention the fact that I was often calling myself stupid when I made mistakes. I wasn't even aware of it. But when you start to listen to yourself and other moms, you realize how, as a group, we can talk to ourselves in ways we would never talk to our kids. And "our own criticisms are the ones that hurt most," says Jerilyn Brownstein, MSW.

The other day, I was on the sideline of my daughter's soccer game when a flustered mom ran up with her kid. They were late for the game because they had just come from gymnastics. "Sorry. I'm a bad mommy. I forgot your soccer shirt for the team picture," the mom said as she frantically changed her daughter out of her leotard. I couldn't help myself. "No, you're not," I responded. "You're just a human being who forgot to bring a soccer shirt."

"Most of us talk to ourselves—narrating our success and failures—all day," says psychotherapist Sarah Best. Psychologists call this "self-talk," and it's very easy for it to veer into negative commentary. That's human. Best recommends listening to the way you talk to yourself and, when you find that you're beating yourself up with your words, evaluate their truth.

If you fed your child nuggets and old celery sticks for dinner one night, are you really a "terrible mother"? Or was it just a busy day and you were tired and needed a quick dinner and an early bedtime? Think about what you would say if your friend told you the same story. Then reframe the way you are judging yourself in that moment.

Just like you work hard to respect your child and help her develop a strong sense of self, you can do the same for you. You're raising a mother at the same time that you are raising a child.

SHOWING YOURSELF COMPASSION

"As mothers, we can get so focused on caring for this other being and you get down on yourself and criticize yourself every time you do something that is not up to your standards," says Kristin Neff, PhD, author of *Self-Compassion: The Proven Power of Being Kind to Yourself* and associate professor of human development and culture at the University of Texas at Austin. "What self-compassion does is embrace the fact that we are imperfect and it's really okay."

Neff—who pioneered the field of self-compassion—is quick to differentiate it from self-esteem. Self-esteem involves a value judgment about how you are being as a mother or as a person. Neff focuses her work on how you *treat* yourself in all the small moments of the day. "Anytime you are facing an emotional struggle or are feeling bad or anxious, treating yourself kindly and with support is a powerful coping mechanism," says Neff.

Most of the people who attend Neff's Mindful Self-Compassion workshops are moms, many with older kids who have special needs. (Neff has a son who is autistic, and she has written about how self-compassion has helped her cope with the emotional struggles she faces raising him.) "There are a couple of moms who come up to me at every workshop and say that they wish they had known about self-compassion when their child was young, how it has really helped them cope with the challenges of being a parent."

"Getting a massage, eating healthy, seeing friends," says Neff. "You can't do those things in the very challenging moments of parenting, but you can practice self-compassion in those moments."

WAYS TO PRACTICE SELF-COMPASSION:

Touch Yourself in a Soothing Way

"All mammals have three universal triggers of the caregiver system," says Neff. "Warmth, gentle touch, and soothing vocalizations." When you gently put your hands on your heart or your face and say some soothing words to yourself, your parasympathetic nervous system kicks in. Your body feels soothed, and you can think more clearly about the decisions you want to make. "People are always amazed at how powerful it is," says Neff. "It seems really touchy-feely, but there are physiological underpinnings to it."

Speak to Yourself Kindly

In difficult moments, say a kind phrase to yourself (out loud or in your head), such as "This is suffering" or "I'm feeling stress." Then follow that thought with the acknowledgment that we all experience these moments. Neff suggests phrases such as "Other people feel this way" or "I'm not alone." And finally, put your hand on your heart, touching yourself gently and offer yourself comfort in the form of a phrase such as "May I be kind to myself," "May I forgive myself," or "May I accept myself the way I am."

Try Meditation

Cultivate goodwill and compassion toward yourself and others by trying "loving-kindness meditation" in which you wish peace and health to yourself as you breathe in and the same to others as you breathe out. Neff has a good one on her website, self-compassion.org. Another simple meditation is "affectionate breathing," which Neff recommends doing every day. Pay attention to each breath. As you breathe out, let go of feelings you don't need anymore, and as you breathe in, notice how each breath is nourishing you. Do this with a gentle rocking motion that follows the rising and falling of your breath. "Think of your breath as a friend that is always there for you," says Neff.

Give Yourself Appreciation

While it's powerful to be compassionate to yourself when you make a mistake or are struggling, it's equally important to recognize yourself for all the things you do that are worth appreciating. One way to do this is to keep a journal by your bed and jot down a few things you did that day that you feel good about. You can also "notice anything you are struggling with and write down words of compassion, support, and friendliness to yourself," says Neff.

All these exercises "prime your brain to habitually react that way when times are difficult," says Neff. "When a challenging situation comes up or you make a mistake, it will help you keep an attitude of benevolence and goodwill toward yourself."

Do It for the Kids!

Once again, you alone are worth all the self-compassion you can cultivate, but if you need the motivation or just want to know another benefit, know that you will help your kids develop self-compassion by modeling it for them.

Your kids are "one of the biggest reasons to cultivate a loving mind-set to yourself," says Neff, who has been researching the effect of mirror neurons—neurons that fire in your brain as a result of seeing another person's emotion. It's part of the system that helps us develop empathy as a species. "Whenever I get ramped up, my son will get upset too," says Neff. "And when I show myself self-compassion, he will calm down."

"Anytime you make a mistake or blow it, it's a really great opportunity to model self-compassion," says Neff. "You can say to yourself, 'Gosh, I was stressed,' and model owning your mistakes at the same time that you are not beating yourself up about it. In a way, you can't fail. It's a kind of safety net. There's a teacher in Scotland who says the goal of practice is to be a compassionate mess. If your goal as a mother is to be a compassionate mess, you can achieve it."

Been There, Done That: Moms Talk About Being Kind to Themselves

Forgiving myself is hard. Haven't quite figured that one out just yet.   —JEANNINE, BOSTON, MASSACHUSETTS

I usually talk about it with my husband, and he's pretty good at boosting me up. I definitely haven't mastered doing it for myself.   —KRISTEN, SAN FRANCISCO, CALIFORNIA

I have to forgive myself because nobody else can.
—DAGMAR, ATLANTA, GEORGIA

Guess what? Those were the only quotes moms gave me about being kind to themselves. Looks like we all need to work on this!

Good for Her, but Not for Me

There's a really good Amy Poehler quote about Maya Rudolph," says psychotherapist Sarah Best. "Maya Rudolph had two home births, and Amy Poehler's quote was, 'Good for her! Not for me,' which I think is just a wonderful way to think about birth and motherhood in general. There are lots of choices that are good for her but not for me. If there were one way to do it, we would have figured it out by now."

TO FEEL COMPETITIVE IS TO BE HUMAN

Given the high stakes of parenting we have already discussed, all the options and opinions laid before you, and the fact that you are likely very new to this, comparing yourself to others and feeling competitive is an understandable response.

"When we're in territory where things are scary and new, and we feel unsure about how we're doing it and whether we are doing it right *and* we really care about it, one of the ways that we can reassure ourselves is to take a dogmatic position," says Best. "If you are talking to a group of moms, the dogma will definitely show up. The co-sleepers, for instance, might seem so sure and passionate in their support of co-sleeping. But the baby-in-his-own-room-from-week-two crew seems just as sure, because in any group's fervor, there is an element of reinforcing their choices for themselves."

"The effort to not feel that competition can be hard," says Best. "Sometimes it can help to just acknowledge, 'I'm feeling really competitive with this person right now and that's okay,'" says Best. "We really want to do a good job and are figuring things out as we go. It makes total sense—and isn't a moral failing—if we find ourselves feeling competitive (or defensive or envious) around issues that make us realize we feel less sure than we'd like to be."

BUILD A SUPPORTIVE COMMUNITY

"The most important thing we can do to build our confidence as moms is to surround ourselves with people in our lives who help us feel like good parents," says author Carla Naumburg. And that doesn't necessarily mean only having parent friends who share your specific parenting choices, but people who support you in making choices that are good for you and your family.

"It can be easy to fall into a group of mom friends because you happen to have taken the same 'Mommy and Me' classes or share the same schedule," says Naumburg. "I had one mom friend and every time I came away from hanging out with her, I'd think, *Oh my god, I'm screwing up my parenting.* There was something about our interaction that was triggering for me in that way."

"A therapist once said to me, 'It's not about whether you and a spouse are going to fight; it's about how you fight and how you make up,'" says parenting coach Dana Rosenbloom. In other words, it's good to have parent friends who can respect and be open to your approaches, even as they remain comfortable and open about theirs.

DON'T COMPARE YOUR INSIDES TO OTHER PEOPLE'S OUTSIDES

"Research shows that when you compare yourself [negatively] to others, it decreases your well-being," says life coach Debra Levy. "That's where Facebook and social media can be an emotional killer."

"Yeah, it can be a major confidence eroder when you feel that other moms are training for marathons, baking their kids brownies, and signing them up for soccer," agrees Naumburg. But it's important to remember that "you get to see people at their very best on Instagram, and that's what you compare your world to," adds Carrie Bruno, IBCLC, creator of the Mama Coach in Calgary, Canada.

"There's this general feeling of 'All these moms have it so together,'" says psychologist Kate Bieger. "With absolute confidence, I tell every mom who is struggling, 'No matter what another mom looks like, the ones who look like they have it the most together are the ones who are struggling the most behind the scenes.'"

LISTEN TO YOURSELF

"A lot of parenting is quieting the cultural noise all around us that's interfering with our own judgments of how to care for our children," says Ayelet Kaznelson, an internationally board-certified lactation consultant in New York City. "There's a lot of information around—from family and friends—that's not necessarily accurate," says Kaznelson. What does she recommend in moments of comparison or self-doubt? Ask yourself, "Is it working for you?"

REMEMBER HOW MUCH WE VALUE DIVERSITY?!

From the beginning of the daycare search to the college application process, there is one word everyone throws about as the watermark of a progressive society—*diversity*. But somehow that appreciation flies out the window when it comes to motherhood and parenthood.

Many of us either watch other moms wondering why our approach is not more like theirs or lauding ourselves for having a different (read: superior) approach. Lost in that binary proposition is the beautiful fact that there are all kinds of mothers on the planet and all kinds of ways to raise kids—and if you can tap into that appreciation, that's living the value of diversity.

"When I was trained, one of the best things I was ever taught was that each family has its own culture," says Rosenbloom. "If families can honor that about their family, then they can take all these competing ideas with a grain of salt as they learn what their needs—and their children's needs—are."

LET OTHER PEOPLE ENRICH YOUR KID

You do not have to be—nor can you be—all things to your child. You have brought a person into the *world*, and that world is filled with all different kinds of people who can offer your child things you cannot or do not want to. What a relief!

When my older daughter was three, she wanted to stop and close every single wrought iron gate on our Brooklyn brownstone street. I had no time or patience for that. But you know who did? My mother-in-law. When she took care of my daughter, they would take an hour to go one block. I'd have pulled all my hair out and yelled at my poor toddler five minutes into the slow, completely present walks they took, but I didn't have to. I could hurry my toddler along when we were out and about and let my mother-in-law Zen out with her on the other days. (Thank you, DG!)

In my other job as editorial director of the Seleni Institute, I edited a terrific piece by Rosenbloom that spoke to this exact idea—that your child's community can enrich your child's life in ways you can't or don't want to.

Allowing your child time to interact with other adults is a wonderful learning opportunity for them. The caregiver who sings can teach your child about melody. The grandparent who loves to bike ride gives your child the ability to experience outings in a new way. All of these moments enhance your child's development, flexibility, and resilience. We'll never all be good at the same thing, and that's a good thing. Children grow by interacting and relating to others, especially people with areas of expertise that are different from yours. Just like we do, our kids benefit from new relationships and exposures to new experiences.

In fact, Rosenbloom put it so well, I'm going to close this section out with her wise words:

Parenting isn't one size fits all. How boring would it be if we all parented the same way? And how quickly would we lose the wonderful differences between people if they were all raised with the same experiences? Through experimentation and reflection and with good support, parents come up with their own answers and figure out the best way for themselves, their individual family, and their unique child. So ask questions. Try new skills. Forgive yourself when it doesn't work out, and appreciate when others succeed where you did not. It's not easy, but I give you permission to release yourself from self-doubt and learn to love the parent you are becoming every day.

Can I get an amen?

Been There, Done That: Moms Talk About Comparisons in Motherhood

---

Stand by your chosen path and your decisions with confidence, but also don't be afraid to ask for help if you're not sure which path to take. Remember all moms are doing their best, so try hard not to judge. There are many ways to get to the same place.

—HOLLY, BROOKLYN, NEW YORK

Do not compare yourself to others, ever. You are you; your baby and your family are unique. Trust that you are doing the best you can.   —SARA, ATLANTA, GEORGIA

It's sometimes hard not to be judgmental or feel "superior" to another parent. Hopefully I don't vocalize that if I do feel it. What helps me is to try to put myself into that person's position. It's easy to think, I'd do it differently, *until you're faced with the situation directly.*

—DAGMAR, ATLANTA, GEORGIA

I remind myself that none of us have it all together, even if some moms are better at pretending they do. I try not to compare myself to other moms, and I try not to compare my kid to other kids. We have made every facet of living a competition for ourselves and our kids. It's exhausting. All of us have completely different journeys and experiences.

—JENNIFER, ATLANTA, GEORGIA

Honestly, the thing that helps me most when I compare myself to moms I think of as better than I am is when they acknowledge their weaknesses and failings. That sounds terrible to admit, but it kind of cracks their perfect veneer and gives me perspective.

—JULIE, SAN FRANCISCO, CALIFORNIA

Instagram can go suck it.

—BRANDY, CHICAGO, ILLINOIS

I usually try to praise moms when I see something I like. I believe we should have a community that brings us up instead of pushing each other down.

—PATTY, DECATUR, GEORGIA

You Are Good Enough

Once upon a time, there was a pediatrician and psychoanalyst in England named Donald Winnicott. He believed in a great many good things, such as the value of empathy and imagination, that play was a vital part of emotional well-being for adults and children, and that "the foundations of health are laid down by the ordinary mother in her ordinary loving care of her own baby."

Winnicott wanted to convey to women that they shouldn't worry too much about what "experts" or others had to say about childcare. "Unthinking people will often try to teach you how to do the things which you can do better than you can be taught to do them," he told mothers during a BBC broadcast talk in 1950.

Sure, the overemphasis over the years on a mother's role as primary in a child's development has had its share of problems (just see "Beware the Cult of Perfect Motherhood" on page 317), but, considering that Winnicott was a male in an academic and medical world in the post–World War II era, he was pretty damn progressive. At a time when much of the mental health establishment was warning that mothers were threatening national security by raising neurotic sons due to their own neuroses, Winnicott cut through that noise with the concept of the "good enough mother."

After watching and researching thousands of babies with their mothers, Winnicott discerned that when mothers are "ordinarily" attuned to—and meet—their babies needs in the big categories (being held, fed, and loved), their babies gain confidence that the world is a safe place. Then, over time, "good enough mothers" separate from their children and fail them in small ways—by not meeting their every need, not fixing every problem—so that the children learn resilience, the ability to self-soothe, and faith that they can fix things themselves.

"Winnicott wasn't saying give up on perfection because your kids will be okay with good enough," says author Carla Naumburg, PhD. "He was saying good enough is *good* for your kids."

OUR JOB IS NOT TO MAKE OUR KIDS HAPPY

"The most problematic message that moms are getting is that we are responsible for our child's happiness and that if our kid isn't happy, it's because we haven't worked hard enough," says Naumburg. "This is a recipe for failure."

The flip side of that is that "if we do everything right, our kids will grow up to be happy, healthy doctors and Peace Corps workers," says Naumburg. "That's not true. There are a million moving parts. There are people who come from warm, nurturing families who struggle their whole lives, and people who come from really dysfunctional families that do just fine.

Your child's happiness is not an indication of how good of a parent you are."

RESILIENCE IS THE GOAL—FOR EVERYONE

As your children will tell you a million times before the age of six, life is "not fair." Things go wrong. People get hurt, disappointed, angry. Accidents happen. Life is messy, and the greatest gifts you can give yourself and your child are the tools to tolerate the difficult parts. That is what your child is busy doing as he grows, and if you try to step in and smooth over all the bumps, avoid all the pitfalls, you will not only drive yourself crazy but you will deny your child the opportunity to learn that he can cope in the face of adversity and move through it.

"An important part of kids growing up is to have emotional stability and be able to function in the world," says Kate Bieger. "We want them to come up against disappointment. Our job as parents is not to make things easy or always good. It's about teaching our kids how to meet the difficult moments and the struggles."

Or, as Naumburg wrote on her *Psych Central* blog, "Building our children's resilience is the gift of the good enough mother." And I would add to that a second gift—building our own resilience.

Winnicott's good enough mother is a real person who has ambivalence about motherhood. She can resent it, even hate it at times, and she has her own interests and needs to attend to. And, in doing so, she gives her children the space to find their own way.

SOMETHING HAS GOT TO GIVE—AND THAT'S
A GOOD THING

Not only do your children benefit from small failures and learning how to bounce back, but you do too. The Cult of Perfect Motherhood, plus the general pressures of work, family, and life will pile a list of demands on you that no one person could possibly meet. And even if you could, would you want to? What would that life look like?

"The reality is that when you are a parent, something's got to give," says Nitzia Logothetis, founder and chairwoman of the Seleni Institute. "If I could help women in only one way, it would be to help them understand it's okay to just be good enough, because what you are considering is your mediocre self is probably amazing."

"I remember watching this video where they interviewed a bunch of mothers about how they felt about themselves as mothers, and then they asked the kids what they felt about their mothers," says Bieger. "It's such a tearjerker, because the moms were so self-critical and the kids went on and on about how great their moms were. As moms, we are often looking at one wrong moment instead of seeing all these different things that our children are getting from us."

Stop and look at the big picture. What really matters to you and your kids, and what can you let go of in order to have more space in your life for those things? What would it look like to be good enough for your kids and good enough for you? Can you try it out? I will if you will.

Been There, Done That: Moms Talk About Being "Good Enough"

If my kids are loved, educated, and alive at the end of the day, I have done well.   —AMANDA, PORTLAND, OREGON

I'm pretty good with the mom I am to the children I have.
—JEANNINE, BOSTON, MASSACHUSETTS

I am filling my son's basic needs and then some. He has a much better setup in life than I had as a small child. Part of being good enough is showing him he has to try things on his own, fall down and skin his knees, make mistakes, enjoy successes when he tries things.
—SUSAN, DECATUR, GEORGIA

I try to remember that the most important thing is making a child feel loved and secure.
—NICOLE, BROOKLYN, NEW YORK

As they've gotten older and seem to have turned out all right, I do, in fact, feel like I've been good enough! I didn't always feel this way, especially when I only had one colicky baby and thought it was all my fault, but now, almost sixteen years in—with two thoughtful, kind, and curious kids—I feel like they've turned out okay!
—MARGARET, BROOKLYN, NEW YORK

Being Strong As a Mother

*Strength (n) definition 2.1: "The emotional or mental qualities
necessary in dealing with difficult or distressing situations."*
—OXFORD ENGLISH DICTIONARY

What does *strong* mean to you?

Is strong not using medication through a very painful thirty-hour labor? Is it knowing that you would like pain relief in labor and asking for it? Is strong never complaining? Is it admitting when things are hard? Is strong feeling a little better today than you felt yesterday? Is it the mother in line at the grocery store who calmly says no to her toddler's incessant whining for candy? Is strong asking for help? Is it struggling but keeping it together? Is strong never having to ask for help and being able to do it on your own? Is it admitting when you made a mistake? Is strong being right? Is strong creating a village that can help you? Is strong putting your children first? Is it putting yourself first? Or is it a combination of the two? Is strong never letting them see you sweat? Is it being physically strong? Has this book changed the idea you have of what strength entails? Are you drawing a blank?

Here are some definitions of strong quickly compiled for me by ye olde Google.

- "Having the power to move heavy weights or perform other physically demanding tasks"
- "Able to perform a specified action well and powerfully"
- "Exerting great force"
- "Likely to succeed because of sound reasoning or convincing evidence"
- "Possessing skills and qualities that create a likelihood of success"
- "Powerfully affecting the mind, senses, or emotions"
- "Able to withstand great force or pressure"
- "Very intense"
- "Not soft or muted; clear or prominent"
- "Forceful and extreme, especially excessively or inappropriately so"

I think those are apt descriptions of the experience of motherhood, and many describe the qualities moms possess without even thinking about them.

Some, like "having the power to move heavy weights or perform other physically demanding tasks," is just in the job description. You have already probably spent a great deal of your time as a mom literally (and/or figuratively) carrying a heavy weight and performing "physically demanding tasks."

Others on the list might not be what pops to mind when you think of strength, like "powerfully affecting the mind, senses, or emotions." But if that is not a spot-on definition of motherhood, I don't know what is. And note, it does not characterize "affecting." It's just saying that something strong has the ability to exert great influence over your psychological state. Oh yeah, that's motherhood. The same goes for "very intense." Check.

And what about "likely to succeed because of sound reasoning or convincing evidence" or "possessing skills and qualities that create a likelihood of success"? If you can ignore the word *success* (which is too loaded a term for my taste), these are beautiful little Zen koans that could be very helpful in the inevitable moments of doubt and times when you beat yourself up for what you think you are not doing, or cannot do, as a mom.

If you can slow down in those moments and exhibit self-compassion (see page 335), what a great little discovery you can make—that "sound reasoning" and "convincing evidence" are all around you, that you "got this."

Finally, we arrive at: "forceful and extreme, especially excessively or inappropriately so." *Excessive* or *inappropriate* are words that are usually used to pass negative judgment on something, but they are also words that reflect a cultural norm around behavior. And you already know that my life's work is to soften, deconstruct, ignore, or, at the very best, change the cultural norms around what it means to be a mother, so I love that last one.

I think it will take a whole lot of us being "clear and prominent," "forceful and extreme"—especially "excessively or inappropriately so"—to change the societal perceptions that can keep us from feeling strong as mothers. This certainly applies to political action, but in this book, I am talking about the tiny personal revolutions we are all capable of in our own lives as we decide what it means to be strong as a mother.

Here's my evolving list of what I think being strong as a mother means:

Making an effort to:
- recognize that struggle is normal
- ask for help through it
- surround yourself with people who will support you
- figure out what you need and ask for it
- do the things that build your resilience
- recover from setbacks
- celebrate yourself and recognize all that you do
- open up when things don't feel right
- rely on your partner and others to parent beside you
- show and accept weakness
- forgive yourself
- give yourself the benefit of the doubt
- accept that sometimes you fall down
- know that you will eventually get back up
- understand that mistakes are how you learn
- be present in the journey and process of parenthood
- rest when you need to
- accept yourself for who you are and where you are
- love yourself through all of it

Whatever strength means to you, my wish for you is that you search for it, find it, hold on to it, and pick it back up when you inevitably lose track of it.

Because there is no one on this planet as strong as a mother.

Acknowledgments

I feel like one of those people at the Oscars hastily referring to notes about whom to thank, certain the music will start playing and she will have forgotten someone. So let me start out by saying, if I forgot you but you know how much you have supported me—as a mother and as I wrote this book—know that I deeply appreciate you. I will remember that I forgot you at 3:00 A.M. two nights after this goes to print and be unable to sleep for the rest of the night. Then I will wake up in the morning, follow my own advice, and forgive myself for being human.

With that caveat out of the way, I want to express my deep gratitude for:

My parents, for being what my husband calls *überparents*—giving me everything I needed to have the support, experiences in life, and the confidence to write this book. I learned how to be strong from one of the strongest mothers. (If you don't believe me, just try to "play hardball" with her. She's been "doing it a lot longer than you!") But, seriously, Mom, thank you for leading by feminist example and showing me how to be a strong mother and a strong woman—and Dad, thanks for being a feminist (albeit "not a militant one"), and thank you both so much for—everything.

My husband, for living up to vow number eight and inspiring me—from the moment we met—to take bigger risks than I ever want to, for teaching me what it is to have bald confidence in yourself, and for being my best editor.

My two girls, for their patience as their mom kinda disappeared (physically and metaphorically) for six months to get this book done.

Sarah Best, for being my professional beacon through my career as a maternal mental health writer and editor, for talking with me for hours to help me shape the content of this book, and for reading every word of it to make it better.

Becca Benghiat, for violating the anonymity rules on Park Slope Parents and reaching out to me to ask me to write that first article for the Seleni Institute. Who knew that cup of coffee we had at Deluxe on Seventh Avenue would change my career in the most meaningful way yet? Actually, you might have known, because you're like that.

George and Nitzia Logothetis, for having the vision and heart to create an organization dedicated to strengthening mothers and their families—the Seleni Institute—and for putting so much of themselves into creating it.

To all the clinicians and staff of Seleni with whom I have worked over the past five years. You have taught me more than I can ever repay, and your dedication inspires me.

Samantha Meltzer-Brody, for being a continually accessible

and warm expert source who is surprisingly available given how busy she is and her achievements in the field of maternal mental health. In particular for taking the time, on short notice, to read and review my entire section on perinatal mood and anxiety disorders to make sure it reflected the most current scientific understanding.

Carla Naumburg, for giving me some great tools to take care of myself and for being my virtual soul mate. I'm so glad we are going to finally meet in person!

Sarah Hrdy, PhD, for patiently explaining important evolutionary concepts to me and for deepening and broadening my understanding of motherhood through her books and conversation.

Lauren Smith Brody, for being so generous with her knowledge, resources, and network while helping me get this book out there.

Mara Acel-Green, for being an awesome support for families and for having a delicious brainstorming dinner with me early on.

All the clinicians and activists on the front lines of women's mental health, especially those that shared their work with me for this book.

My psychotherapist, DD, for being exactly what I needed.

My psychiatrist, MK, for helping me truly understand the biochemical nature of mental health and that it is no different than physical health.

Graeme Seabrook, for giving me one of the most inspiring interviews I had for this book and for serving as an informal consigliere as I approached deadline.

All the women who took the time to fill out my surveys and honestly share their experiences. Your words will matter more than any of mine in this book. A particular thanks to my local moms' Facebook group for your patience with my endless posts and requests for help—both professionally and personally. You guys rock.

Nicole Allen, for spending hours cultivating and indulging my children's imaginations while I hammered away on the keys to get this book done and for being a shining example of the value of letting other people share in the raising of your kids.

Deborah Gilmartin, for a wonderful, imaginative week of "Nan Camp" as I turned into the home stretch, and for demonstrating for my daughters and me the value of quiet, steady strength.

My brother, for being a feminist uncle to his two strong nieces and for talking me down from several anxiety ledges.

Meg Watson and Graham Kirkland, for inspiring me to take writers' weekends and for watching my kids when I did—and also for just being awesome.

Diana Anders, for giving me the safest space to share all my feelings and for being the nonjudgmental friend I want this book to be for my readers.

Ariel Flavin, for growing up with me as a mom and helping me be more compassionate to myself along the way and for reading my book and giving me the best review anyone could ask for (and some really great advice for making it better). Let's never "feel bad about ourselves again!"

MeiMei Fox, for being a wonderful lifelong friend and

professional beacon in the world of book writing and for giving me so many great quotes!

Laurel Snyder and Kate Tuttle, for being my writing buddies and for their insightful feedback and friendship.

K. J. Dell'Antonia, for sharing precious book publicity resources.

Josh Guerrieri and Ethan Duff and the entire staff at Fit-Wit, for showing me that moving my body every day feels great and can change everything. You know it is not an exaggeration to say you guys are changing lives!

Ashleigh Henneberger, for helping me cut pages when I thought there was nothing else I could possibly cut.

My editor, Nichole Argyres, for her unwavering support and comforting guidance. I always feel better when I get off the phone with you! Have you thought about going into the mental health field?

Courtney Littler, my associate editor, for the best eye for cuts in the biz!

Lisa Davis, production editor; Eric Gladstone, production manager; Emily Mahon, jacket designer; Michelle McMillian, book designer; and Sara and Chris Ensey, copyeditors. You guys make me look good!

Kirsten Wolf, esq. at Wolf Literary Services, for keeping it all on the up-and-up!

And all the people I forgot. Thank you.

Appendix

Super Helpful Resources and Places to Find Support

ABUSE (PHYSICAL OR VERBAL)

The National Domestic Violence Hotline, 800-799-7233

Domesticshelters.org (searchable database of shelters nationwide)

Asian Task Force Against Domestic Violence, 617-338-2355, atask.org

ADOPTION

The Center for Adoption Support and Education's Directory of Adoption Competent Professionals, adoptionsupport.org/

North American Council on Adoptable Children, Parent Groups database, nacac.org/connect/parent-group/

North American Council on Adoptable Children's Self-Care: Barriers and Basics for Foster/Adoptive Parents, nacac.org/resource/self-care-barriers-adoptive-parents/

BIRTH

Preparation

DONA (international certification for Doulas), dona.org

Birthing from Within, birthingfromwithin.com

Postpartum Support International, Birth and Postpartum Doulas, postpartum.net/get-help/birth-and-postpartum-doulas/

Survivors of Sexual Assault

Pregnancy to Parenting: A Guide for Survivors of Sexual Abuse,
   angelfire.com/moon2/jkluchar1995/abuse.html
*Survivor Moms: Women's Stories of Birthing, Mothering and Healing After
   Sexual Assault*, by Mickey Sperlich and Julia S. Seng

Traumatic

Solace for Mothers, solaceformothers.org
The Birth Trauma Association, birthtraumaassociation.org.uk
Trauma and Birth Stress, tabs.org.nz
Birth Story Medicine, birthingfromwithin.com/pages/birth-story
   -medicine

Breastfeeding

Breastfeeding Made Simple, breastfeedingmadesimple.com
The Boob Group podcast, newmommymedia.com/the-boob-group/
International Lactation Consultant Association, Find a Lactation Con-
   sultant, ilca.org/why-ibclc/falc
Kelly Mom, kellymom.com
La Leche League International, llli.org
Breastfeeding Solutions App for your phone

Adoptive and Non-Birth Parents:

Breastfeeding without Birthing, sweetpeabreastfeeding.com/resources.html
*Breastfeeding Without Birthing: A Breastfeeding Guide for Mothers
   Through Adoption, Surrogacy, and Other Special Circumstances*, by
   Alyssa Schnell

After Breast or Nipple Surgery

BFAR, bfar.org

D-MER

D-MER.org

Moms of Color

Black Women Do Breastfeed, blackwomendobreastfeed.org

Pumping

Work, Pump, Repeat: The New Mom's Survival Guide to Breastfeeding and Going Back to Work, by Jessica Shortall

Breastfeeding and Exclusively Pumping Group Support, facebook.com /groups/335090556210/?ref=group_browse_new

Survivors of Sexual Assault

Survivor Moms: Women's Stories of Birthing, Mothering and Healing After Sexual Assault, by Mickey Sperlich and Julia S. Seng

PTSD and Breastfeeding, angelfire.com/moon2/jkluchar1995/breast feeding.html

Trans Families

Birthing and Breast or Chestfeeding Trans People and Allies, facebook .com/groups/TransReproductiveSupport/?ref=group_browse_new

DADS

See "Fathers"

DOMESTIC VIOLENCE

See "Abuse (Physical or Verbal)"

EATING DISORDERS / BODY IMAGE

Eating Disorder Referral and Information Center, edreferral.com

National Eating Disorders Association Helpline, 800-931-2237

FATHERS (RESOURCES AND GROUPS)

Postpartum Dads, postpartumdads.org

Postpartum men, postpartummen.com

Postpartum Support International, Dads Chat with an Expert, post partum.net/chat-with-an-expert/chat-with-an-expert-for-dads

Boot Camp for New Dads, bootcampfornewdads.org

The Good Men Project, goodmenproject.com/category/families

Men Excel, Advice for New Dads, menexcel.com/advice-for-new -dads

Just4Dads.org, just4dads.org/supportgroups

The Seleni Institute, 212-939-7200, seleni.org/advice-support/topic
      /fatherhood
Meetup.com (search for "fatherhood" or "dads' groups")
Fatherly.com

FORMULA-FEEDING

*Bottled Up: How the Way We Feed Babies Has Come to Define Motherhood,
      and Why It Shouldn't,* by Suzanne Barston
Fearless Formula Feeder, fearlessformulafeeder.com; on Facebook,
      facebook.com/FearlessFormulaFeeder
Pediatrician Chad Hayes' website, chadhayesmd.com/formula
The Bump Formula-Feeding Forums, forums.thebump.com/categories
      /formula-feeding

FUSSY BABIES

The Fussy Baby Site, thefussybabysite.com
Fussy Baby Network, 888-431-BABY, erikson.edu/fussy-baby-network/
The Period of Purple Crying, purplecrying.info
The Happiest Baby on the Block, by Harvey Karp

HIGH-RISK PREGNANCY

See "Pregnancy: Complications / High Risk"

HYPEREMESIS GRAVIDARUM

Help HER: Hyperemesis Education Research, helpher.org

LGBTQ FAMILIES

Lesbian, Gay, Bisexual and Transgender National Hotline, 888-843-
      4564
Lambda Legal resources for parental protection, lambdalegal.org/know
      -your-rights/article/planning-protecting-your-children
Lambda Legal state-by-state guide to laws about adoption or second-
      parent adoption, lambdalegal.org/states-regions/in-your-state
Lambda Legal Help Desk, lambdalegal.org/helpdesk
National Queer and Trans Therapists of Color Directory, nqttcn.com
      /directory

MEDICATION

During Pregnancy and Breastfeeding

The Infant Risk Center, 806-352-2519, infantrisk.com

Motherisk Pregnancy Helpline, 877-439-2744

Mother to Baby, 866-626-6847, text: 855-999-3525, mothertobaby.org

APPS

MommyMeds (run by the Infant Risk Center)

LactMed

BOOKS

The Complete Guide to Medications During Pregnancy and Breastfeeding, by
   Carl Weiner and Kate Rope

Medications and Mother's Milk, by Thomas Hale

MATERNAL FETAL MEDICINE

Society for Maternal Fetal Medicine directory (you can search by zip
   code), www.smfm.org/members

MENTAL HEALTH ORGANIZATIONS AND PROFESSIONALS

Finding a Mental Health Professional (General)

Psychology Today's Find a Therapist tool (you can search by specialty),
   psychologytoday.com

GoodTherapy.org

The American Psychological Association's Psychologist Locator (you
   can search by specialty), locator.apa.org

The Anxiety and Depression Association of America, treatment.adaa
   .org

International OCD Foundation, iocdf.org/find-help

Association for Behavioral and Cognitive Therapies, findcbt.org/xFAT

National Alliance for Mental Illness Helpline, 800-950-6264

Mental Health America, mentalhealthamerica.net

American Society on Clinical Psychopharmacology, ascpp.org/resources
   /psychopharmacologist-database/find-a-psychopharmacologist
   -database/

Adoptive families

The Center for Adoption Support and Education's Directory of Adoption Competent Professionals, adoptionsupport.org/

Couples

American Association for Marriage and Family Therapy, therapist locator.net

Fathers

The Seleni Institute, 212-939-7200, seleni.org

Grief

Psychology Today, Find a Grief Therapist, therapists.psychologytoday .com/grief/

The Seleni Institute, 212-939-7200, seleni.org

Association for Death Educators and Counseling, adec.org

The Center for Complicated Grief, complicatedgrief.columbia.edu

Postpartum Support International, Loss and Grief in Pregnancy and Postpartum, postpartum.net/get-help/loss-grief-in-pregnancy -postpartum

LGBTQ

National Queer and Trans Therapists of Color Directory, nqttcn.com

National Alliance on Mental Illness, nami.org/Find-Support/LGBTQ

Association for Lesbian, Gay, Bisexual, and Transgender Issues in Counseling, algbtic.org/therapist-resource-listing.html

The Association of LGBTQ Psychiatrists, aglp.memberclicks.net/simple -search

Lesbian, Gay, Bisexual, and Transgender National Hotline, 888-843- 4564, glbtnationalhelpcenter.org

Low-Cost Options

Open Path Psychotherapy Collective, openpathcollective.org

University or other academic institutions with counseling training programs that offer reduced rates for therapy provided by practitioners in training

Search for community clinics offered by your city or county
Group therapy

Military
Postpartum Support International, PSI Support for Military Families,
    postpartum.net/get-help/psi-support-for-military-families

People of Color
Therapy for Black Girls Therapist Directory, therapyforblackgirls.com
    /therapist-directory
Mental Resources for Women of Color, compiled by the Postpartum
    Mama, postpartummama.org/2017/01/mental-health-resources
    -women-color.html
Postpartum Progress, Black Mental Health Providers List, postpartum
    progress.com/black-mental-health-providers-list
Tessera Collective, Find a Therapist, tesseracollective.org/find-a
    -therapist
National Association for Mental Illness guide to finding a culturally
    competent provider, nami.org/Find-Support/Diverse-Communities
African American Therapists Directory, africanamericantherapists.com
Association of Black Psychologists' directory, abpsi.org/find-psychologists
Akoma Counseling Concepts (DC area), akomacounselingconcepts.com
Black Girl+Mental Health blog, blackgirlmentalhealth.tumblr.com
Tessera Collective private support group on Facebook, facebook.com
    /tesseracollective/
Redefine Enough, 5 Mental Health Podcasts by Therapists of Color,
    redefineenough.com/blog/5-mental-health-podcasts-by-therapists
    -of-color
National Asian American Pacific Islander Mental Health Association,
    naapimha.org
Together Empowering Asian Minds (TEAM), teamasianminds.org
National Association of Mental Illness Latino Mental Health, nami
    .org/Find-Support/Diverse-Communities/Latino-Mental-Health
Mental Health America Latino/Hispanic Communities and Mental
    Health, mentalhealthamerica.net/issues/latinohispanic-communities
    -and-mental-health

American Society of Hispanic Psychiatry, americansocietyhispanicpsy
chiatry.com/

Perinatal Mood and Anxiety Disorders

National Resources

Postpartum Support International Warmline, 800-944-4773, postpar
tum.net

Postpartum Support International National Database of Support,
postpartum.net/get-help/locations

The Postpartum Stress Center in Rosemont, Pennsylvania, 610-525-
7527 postpartumstress.com

The Seleni Institute in Manhattan, 212-939-7200 seleni.org

Postpartum Support International, Intensive Perinatal Psych Treatment in the U.S., postpartum.net/professionals/intensive-perinatal
-psych-treatment-in-the-us

Postpartum Progress nationwide list of providers, postpartumprogress
.com/womens-mental-health-treatment-programs-specialists-us
-canada-australia

Postpartum Progress nationwide list of support groups, postpartum
progress.com/ppd-support-groups-in-the-u-s-canada

California

MemorialCare Center for Mental Health and Wellness at Community
Medical Center Long Beach, memorialcare.org/services/mental
-health/mental-health-community-hospital-long-beach/perinatal
-mood-and-anxiety

El Camino Hospital Maternal Outreach Mood Services, elcamino
hospital.org/services/mental-health/specialty-programs/maternal
-outreach-mood-services

Huntington Hospital Postpartum Care, huntingtonhospital.org/Our
-Services/Womens-Health/Obstetrics/Postpartum

Women's Reproductive Health Center at UC San Diego Hospital, health
.ucsd.edu/specialties/psych/clinic-based/reproductive-mental
-health

Georgia

Postpartum Support International Georgia chapter, psiga.org

Illinois

Alexian Brothers Health System, Perinatal Intensive Outpatient Program, alexianbrothershealth.org/abbhh/ourservices/perinatal-IOP

Women's Mental Health and Reproductive Psychiatry at the University of Illinois at Chicago, 312-996-2200

Feinberg School of Medicine, Women's Behavioral Health, psychiatry .northwestern.edu/specialties/womens-health/index.html

Massachusetts

Strong Roots Counseling in Boston, Massachusetts, 857-304-4025, strongrootscounseling.com

Massachusetts General Hospital Center for Women's Mental Health, womensmentalhealth.org

Michigan

Pine Rest Christian Mental Health Services, 800-678-5500, pinerest .org/resource/postpartum-depression-anxiety

Minnesota

Hennepin County Medical Center Mother Baby Program, hcmc.org /clinics/MotherBabyProgram

New Jersey

The Artemis Center for Guidance, 856-345-2820, artemisguidance.com

Monmouth Medical Center Perinatal Mood and Anxiety Center, 732-923-5573 barnabashealth.org/Monmouth-Medical-Center /Our-Services/Obstetrics-Gynecological-Services/Perinatal-Mood -and-Anxiety-Disorder-Center

New York

The Seleni Institute in Manhattan, seleni.org

Women's Mental Health Consortium (a directory of providers who specialize in perinatal mental health in the Greater New York City area), wmhcny.org/directory

The Motherhood Center of New York City, themotherhoodcenter.com

Northwell Health Perinatal Psychiatry Services, northwell.edu/find -care/services-we-offer/perinatal-services

North Carolina

Center for Women's Mood Disorders at the University of North Carolina at Chapel Hill, med.unc.edu/psych/wmd

Pennsylvania

Drexel University Mother Baby Connections, drexel.edu/cnhp /practices/mother-baby-connections

Allegheny Health Network, Women's Behavioral Health, ahn.org /specialties/womens-health/womens-behavioral-health

Rhode Island

Women & Infants Hospital in Providence, Rhode Island, womenand infants.org

Washington

Swedish Center for Perinatal Bonding and Support, swedish.org /locations/center-for-perinatal-bonding-and-support

Postpartum Psychosis

Action on Postpartum Psychosis (hosts online forum for moms to talk to each other), app-network.org

Postpartum Support International, Postpartum Psychosis, postpartum .net/learn-more/postpartum-psychosis

Postpartum Psychosis Alliance on Facebook, facebook.com /postpartumpsychosisawareness

Postpartum Psychosis Forum on Facebook, facebook.com/groups
/357619024101

A Cheat Sheet to Finding the Right Therapist for You
Questions to ask a potential therapist:
What kind of therapy do you practice?
What is your training and background?
What kind of license do you have?
Do you have specific training in the areas I plan to work on?
What is your experience treating clients working through similar issues?
Do you have experience working with people from my culture and
    background?
How do you determine whether you are a good match for a client?
How do you determine whether therapy is working well or not?
If faith or religion is an important part of your life, ask whether your
    therapist is "faith-sensitive," which means they will respect the role
    that religion plays in your life.

Questions to ask yourself to make sure therapy is working for you:
Do I feel that my therapist is present with me and not rushed or dis-
    tracted?
Do I feel seen and understood by him or her? (Does he or she un-
    derstand me, my cultural background, the issues I am working
    through?)
Do I feel comfortable sharing my experiences?
Do I feel heard and accepted?
Do I feel like we are working together?
Do I feel supported and safe even if we are sometimes discussing dif-
    ficult topics?
Does my therapist make me feel emotionally safe and grounded before
    I leave a session?

**MISCARRIAGE (SEE ALSO "MENTAL HEALTH ORGANIZATIONS
    AND PROFESSIONALS: GRIEF")**
The Seleni Institute, 212-939-7200, www.seleni.org; articles on miscar-
    riage: seleni.org/advice-support/topic/miscarriage

Postpartum Support International, Loss and Grief in Pregnancy and Post-
partum, postpartum.net/get-help/loss-grief-in-pregnancy-postpartum
Through the Heart, throughtheheart.org
Share: Pregnancy and Infant Loss Support, nationalshare.org
Grieve Out Loud, grieveoutloud.org
March of Dimes, Dealing with Your Grief, marchofdimes.org
/complications/dealing-with-your-grief-after-the-death-of-year-ba
by.aspx
Psychology Today Support Group Locator, groups.psychologytoday
.com/us/groups

Pregnancy after miscarriage
Pregnancy After Loss Support, pregnancyafterlosssupport.com

MOMS' GROUPS
Program for Early Parent Support (Seattle, Washington), peps.org
Stroller Warriors, strollerwarriors.com
Meetup.com (you can look for specific groups in your area that are
organized around common experiences such as "Asian American
moms" or "formula-feeding moms" or "working moms")
Mocha Moms (for moms of color), mochamoms.org
MOPS (Christian-focused), mops.org
Healthy Start, mchb.hrsa.gov/maternal-child-health-initiatives/healthy
-start
La Leche League (for women who are breastfeeding) llli.org
International Moms Club on Facebook, facebook.com/International
MOMSClub
The Postpartum Mama, postpartummama.org
Self Care Squad on Facebook, facebook.com/groups/selfcaresquad/

Places to Find Moms' Groups
Where you delivered
Local children's stores often coordinate groups by delivery date
Community centers
Story times at local libraries and bookstores
Fitness classes (especially "Mommy and Me")

Meetup.com

Facebook or another online community

Your religious community

NICU

Hand to Hold, handtohold.org

Hand to Hold, NICU Now Podcast

March of Dimes NICU Family Support, marchofdimes.org
/complications/the-nicu-family-support-program.aspx

Support4NICUParents, support4nicuparents.org

PARENTING BOOKS I LIKE

Baby Meets World, by Nicholas Day

The Ages & Stages series from the Louise Ames, PhD, and the Gesell
Institute. (These are from the '50s and '60s, so there is some gender
stereotyping about parental roles, but the child development
information is timeless and very reassuring. Plus, they are short!
You can just read a few reassuring words before nodding off to bed.)

Parenting in the Present Moment, by Carla Naumburg

Peaceful Parents, Happy Kids, by Laura Markham

The Good Mother Myth, by Avital Norman Nathman

PERINATAL MOOD AND ANXIETY DISORDERS

See "Mental Health Organizations and Professionals"

POSTPARTUM DEPRESSION

See "Mental Health Organizations and Professionals"

PREGNANCY

Support groups

Daily Strength, www.dailystrength.org/group/pregnancy

Psychology Today Support Group Locator, groups.psychologytoday
.com

BabyCenter Online Forums, community.babycenter.com

Complications / High Risk

Sidelines High-Risk Pregnancy Support, 888-447-4754, sidelines.org,
    facebook.com/sidelinessupport

March of Dimes Pregnancy Complications, marchofdimes.org
    /complications/pregnancy-complications.aspx

Preeclampsia Foundation, preeclampsia.org

Society for Maternal Fetal Medicine, smfm.org/women-families

BabyCenter Online Forums, community.babycenter.com

RELATIONSHIPS

The Gottman Institute, gottman.com

American Association for Marriage and Family Therapy, therapist
    locator.net

SEX

American Association of Sexuality Educators, Counselors, and
    Therapists, aasect.org/referral-directory

SEXUAL ASSAULT SURVIVORS

*Survivor Moms: Women's Stories of Birthing, Mothering and Healing After
    Sexual Assault,* by Mickey Sperlich and Julia S. Seng

RAINN (Rape, Abuse, and Incest National Network), Recovering from
    Sexual Violence, rainn.org/recovering-sexual-violence

Pregnancy to Parenting: A Guide for Survivors of Sexual Abuse,
    angelfire.com/moon2/jkluchar1995/abuse.html

SOLO MOMS

ESME, esme.com

Meetup.com (search for "single or solo moms' groups")

STILLBIRTH (SEE ALSO "MENTAL HEALTH ORGANIZATIONS AND
PROFESSIONALS: GRIEF")

Reconceiving Loss, reconceivingloss.com

Return to Zero Center for Healing, returntozerohealingcenter.com

The Seleni Institute, 212-939-7200, seleni.org; articles on stillbirth:
    seleni.org/advice-support/tag/stillbirth

Postpartum Support International, Loss and Grief in Pregnancy and
Postpartum, postpartum.net/get-help/loss-grief-in-pregnancy
-postpartum
Share: Pregnancy and Infant Loss Support, nationalshare.org
Grieve Out Loud, grieveoutloud.org
The TEARS Foundation, thetearsfoundation.org
Psychology Today Support Group Locator, groups.psychologytoday
.com/rms/?tr=Hdr_SubBrand

Pregnancy After Stillbirth
Pregnancy After Loss Support, pregnancyafterlosssupport.com

WORKING
Websites
Mindful Return, mindfulreturn.com
The Fifth Trimester, www.thefifthtrimester.com

Books
*The Fifth Trimester: The Working Mom's Guide to Style, Sanity and Big
Success After Baby,* by Lauren Smith Brody
*Back to Work After Baby: How to Plan and Navigate a Mindful Return
from Maternity Leave*, by Lori Mihalich-Levin
*Here's the Plan: Your Practical, Tactical Guide to Steering Your Career
Through Pregnancy and Parenthood*, by Allyson Downey
*Work, Pump, Repeat: The New Mom's Survival Guide to Breastfeeding and
Going Back to Work*, by Jessica Shortall

Online Working Moms' Groups
Mindful Return, facebook.com/mindfulreturn
Meetup.com (search for "working mom groups" in your area)

Index